Understanding Common Diseases
and
the Value of the Pritikin Eating and
Exercise Program

R. James Barnard, Ph.D.
Distinguished Professor Emeritus
University of California, Los Angeles

Understanding Common Diseases and the Value of the
Pritikin Eating and Exercise Program

Written by: R. James Barnard, Ph.D.
Distinguished Professor Emeritus
University of California, Los Angeles

Printed in the United States of America

First paperback printing: August, 2013

ISBN: 978-0-615-86918-6

CONTENTS

Prologue

This book is about the diseases commonly found in the industrialized countries, including heart disease, hypertension, diabetes, obesity, and dementia/Alzheimer's, and the impact that lifestyle plays in their development. Unfortunately, these problems are also becoming prevalent in the developing countries as they adopt the lifestyle of the Westernized countries. While it is true that genes can play a role in their development (a good example is type 2 diabetes), it is also true that lifestyle can be *more* important.

In recent years, there has been considerable debate on the optimal lifestyle for disease prevention. Several approaches exist, from very low-fat 100 percent vegetarian diets to Mediterranean-style diets high in fat from olive oil and nuts. This book is based primarily on the extensive research, more than 100 scientific publications, conducted on behalf of the Nathan Pritikin Research Foundation supporting the value of the Pritikin Program, which is a combination of exercise and an eating plan rich in whole foods like fruits, vegetables, whole grains, and beans, and limited amounts of lean animal protein. All these foods are naturally very low in fat, salt, sugar, and refined carbohydrates.

While more science is needed to determine unequivocally which lifestyle approach has the best results for most individuals, the research presented in this book makes a considerably strong, evidence-based case for the efficacy of the Pritikin Program. From 1981 up until the printing of this book, the data have consistently proven the value of the Pritikin Eating and Exercise Program in preventing, controlling, or reversing the common diseases of our time, including heart disease, diabetes, and hypertension. Key results include:

- Cardiovascular Disease (heart disease and strokes): Significant reductions in virtually all modifiable risk factors, such as LDL cholesterol, triglycerides, inflammatory markers, and excess weight. (See Chapter 2.)
- Hypertension (high blood pressure): Blood pressure lowered to normal or near-normal levels, and the need for medications reduced or eliminated. (See Chapter 3.)
- Diabetes: Multiple risk factors reduced, blood glucose lowered to normal or near-normal levels, and medications for diabetes reduced or eliminated. (See Chapter 4.)

Further, follow-up studies have proven the Pritikin Program's long-term sustainability, due in part to its allowance of large amounts of satisfying foods. No one ever goes hungry on the Pritikin Program.

Nathan Pritikin believed that if people understood the relationship between lifestyle and disease, they would be more likely to adopt a healthy lifestyle like the Pritikin Program. This book discusses the most recent information on the factors thought to underlie the development of the common health problems and how adopting the Pritikin Eating and Exercise Program might prevent and/or control them by influencing not only well-proven risk factors like cholesterol and blood pressure but also emerging risk factors like inflammatory markers.

The Pritikin Program had its origin in the late 1950s/early 1960s as Nathan Pritikin developed the program to treat himself. In 1958 he was diagnosed with ischemic heart disease based on his EKG response during an exercise stress test. His cholesterol was 280 mg/dL in 1955 at his physical examination. In 1958 he was also diagnosed with cancer (a malignant lymphoma). Having the number one and two killers of men in the U.S., he was given no encouragement from his doctors. There were no treatments for cancer, and cholesterol-lowering drugs and bypass surgery were not available to treat coronary disease at that time. Nathan, however, was not content to just sit around until he died. He started to read the literature to find out what societies around the world *not* suffering major epidemics of heart disease and cancer did that made individuals resistant to these problems. He discovered long before John Robbins wrote his book *Healthy at 100*[1] that societies where heart disease and cancer were essentially nonexistent were physically active and consumed a natural food diet of whole grains, vegetables and fruit with limited amounts of animal protein, sometimes almost vegetarian, and were very low in sodium. He described these findings in his first book *Live Longer Now, the First 100 Years of Your Life*[2] published in 1974. By then he had completely changed his lifestyle. He started taking daily walks and changed his diet by eliminating most – or all – animal products and added salt, and greatly increasing his consumption of whole grains, vegetables and fruit. By 1960 his cholesterol had dropped to 120 mg/dL, and in 1969 it was 112 mg/dL. Eventually, his stress test EKG reverted to normal. Convinced that he had regressed his coronary disease, he advanced from daily walking to jogging.

Feeling that he had discovered the answer to many of the health problems so prevalent in the U.S., he assembled a small group of physicians and opened the Pritikin Longevity Center in Santa Barbara, CA, in 1975. The program included a medical examination (including a stress test), daily exercise in the form of walking in the AM and PM, educational lectures on disease and lifestyle given by Mr. Pritikin, and the Pritikin diet consisting of

---

[1] Robbins, John. Healthy at 100: The Scientifically Proven Secrets of the World's Healthiest and Longest-Lived Peoples. New York: Ballantine Books, 2007.
[2] Pritikin, Nathan, Jon N. Leonard, and Jack L. Hofer. Live Longer Now: The First One Hundred Years of Your Life. New York: Ace, 1974.

six meals each day. The diet was primarily vegetarian with the exception of 2 daily servings of nonfat dairy and animal protein (salmon or turkey breast, 3.5 oz.) once a week. Mr. Pritikin referred to this diet as his regression diet and recommended that individuals should follow this diet until their symptoms (angina or claudication) were no longer present, or medications for hypertension or diabetes were discontinued by physicians. Once individuals lost their symptoms or had their medications discontinued, they were permitted to move to the maintenance diet that permitted up to 3.5 oz. of animal protein daily. In the following years Mr. Pritikin enjoyed a vigorous lifestyle jogging on the beach in the early morning, giving lectures and counseling participants at the Longevity Center, as well as speaking to various professional and medical groups. Nathan succumbed to complications from treatment of his leukemia in 1985. The autopsy conducted following his death reported that his coronary arteries "had no raised plaques and no compromise of the lumens"[3] something very rare for a 69-year-old man in the U.S.

In 1978 the Pritikin Longevity Center moved from Santa Barbara to Santa Monica, CA. The medical group that Mr. Pritikin contracted to provide the medical services for the participants hired me as a consultant to organize and direct an in-house, monitored cardiac rehabilitation program as a majority of the participants in the program at that time were cardiac patients. At about the same time, two physicians in Miami, FL, joined Nathan Pritikin to open the Florida Pritikin Center. Also, that same year Mr. Pritikin and his program were featured on the TV program *60 Minutes*. Today the Pritikin Longevity Center and Spa still offers the Pritikin Program in Florida (www.pritikin.com). The present Pritikin Program is described in Figure 8.2. The core of the Pritikin Program includes daily

---

[3] New England Journal of Medicine, 1985; 313: 52.

exercise and the Pritikin Eating Plan. The diet and exercise aspects of the program are complemented by a comprehensive educational program including stress management lectures. This book is meant to complement the Center's educational program.

I was hired as a consultant to design the exercise rehabilitation program for the Pritikin Center based on my credentials. I received my Ph.D. in the field of exercise physiology from the University of Iowa in 1968 followed by a 3-year postdoctoral fellowship in the Department of Medicine at the UCLA School of Medicine, where I conducted biochemical studies related to exercise. Following my postdoctoral training I was hired as a research cardiologist in the Division of Thoracic Surgery, UCLA School of Medicine. In 1975 I served as Vice-President of the American College of Sports Medicine and was involved in developing the cardiac certification program. When I accepted the position as a consultant to the Pritikin Program, I did so with the understanding that Pritikin would not use my name or university affiliation in any of their materials due to the fact that my colleagues in Thoracic Surgery were well aware of the claims Nathan Pritikin had made about the response to his diet and exercise program and thought he was a quack. Mr. Pritikin claimed that his diet and exercise program could lower cholesterol and triglycerides by 25 percent, relieve angina, and patients could avoid bypass surgery. He also claimed that his program could control hypertension and diabetes without the need for medication, claims that most individuals in the medical profession, including myself, thought were ridiculous.

It wasn't long after I started to work with the Pritikin participants that I realized Mr. Pritikin's claims were correct and that most individuals in the medical community, including myself, were unaware of the value of proper diet and exercise for treating coronary patients. At this point I decided to collect data for publication in the medical literature. Little did I realize how difficult it would be to publish data with the name Pritikin on the manuscript. After having manuscripts rejected by several journals, I finally got up enough courage to tell Mr. Pritikin I thought having his name on the papers, even though it belonged, was a problem in getting the papers published. His response was simple, "Just take my name off of the papers. What is important is that we get the information out to the medical community." The first paper was published in 1981[4] and at that time I decided to devote my entire research program at UCLA to study diet, exercise and disease. Since that first paper I have published over 100 research papers related to the Pritikin Program (Chapter 9). Sixty-some included data collected from Pritikin Program participants and forty-some on animal studies supported by several grants from the National Institutes of Health. Some might question the value of using rodents to study diet, exercise and health, but I would point out that placing rodents on a high-fat, refined-sugar diet (similar to the U.S. diet) and placing them in a cage without any exercise led to obesity, hypertension, insulin resistance, elevated triglycerides, increased blood clotting and increased tumor development, problems common in our society. The research clearly shows that adopting the Pritikin lifestyle can prevent and/or control most of the health problems so common in the Westernized societies, and I encourage individuals to follow the Pritikin eating and exercise program described in Chapter 8.

---

[4] Journal of Cardiac Rehabilitation, 1981; 1: 99.

Chapter 1

Why We Die Too Soon With Such Misery

Ernst Wynder, M.D., founder and past president of the American Health Foundation, once said, "My goal is to die as late in life, as young as possible." Unfortunately, too many people in this country die too early, after months of suffering and distress. Why is this so? It is true that life expectancy in the

> **Among 17 wealthy nations, including Canada, Japan, and much of Western Europe, the U.S. ranked 17th for men and 16th for women in life expectancy.**

United States has increased by about 20 years over the past century, from approximately 55 years to 77 years with women living about 4 years longer than men. Life expectancy is defined as the average number of years any given individual might expect to live. In other words, it is the age at which 50 percent of a given population will die. This means that some will die sooner and some later in life. Although life expectancy has increased steadily over the past century, it is anticipated that this will stop and the present generation of young people will be the first *not* to outlive their parents. This is due to the obesity problem and associated medical conditions that have been well documented in young people today. The latest statistics already show that life expectancy is on the decline in some counties in the south where the obesity problem is the greatest. It is also interesting to note that even though the U.S. spends more money on medicine than any other country, we rank 36th and 33rd in life expectancy for men and women worldwide, according to World Health Organization (WHO) statistics. A 2013 report by two of

America's leading health research institutions, the National Research Council and the Institute of Medicine, found that among 17 wealthy nations, including Canada, Japan, and much of Western Europe, the U.S. ranked 17th for men and 16th for women in life expectancy.[5]

Over the past century, life expectancy did increase overall, but we have seen a major change in the cause of death. In the late 1800s most people died from infectious diseases, pneumonia, influenza, tuberculosis, etc., with less than 15 percent of the deaths due to cardiovascular disease and cancer. Today, the majority of deaths are due to cardiovascular disease (36 percent) and cancer (23 percent).[6] In addition, many individuals suffer from the complications of diabetes such as blindness (retinopathy), kidney failure (nephropathy), nerve damage (neuropathy), amputation, and premature heart disease. Because of the increase in life expectancy over the past century, many have assumed that these common health problems are a result of aging and thus, they have been called degenerative or chronic diseases or in some cases have been blamed on genes. In reality, the premature development of these diseases is largely a direct result of lifestyles, eating habits, lack of regular exercise, and exposure to hazardous chemicals that are so pervasive in our environment.[7] Avoiding these common health problems means more people could achieve the normal human lifespan of approximately 100 years. Lifespan is defined as the age at which 90 percent of the population has died. Although there have been claims of some individuals living to be 130 years or older, these ages have never been scientifically documented. In his

---

[5] National Research Council. U.S. Health in International Perspective: Shorter Lives, Poorer Health. Washington, DC: The National Academies Press, 2013.
[6] Centers for Disease Control and Prevention: Leading Causes of Death. http://www.cdc.gov/nchs/fastats/lcod.htm
[7] Centers for Disease Control and Prevention: Chronic Diseases and Health Promotion. http://www.cdc.gov/chronicdisease/overview/index.htm

fascinating book *Healthy at 100*,[8] John Robbins describes several societies around the globe in the 1980s that had achieved survival to the normal lifespan of 100 years while being healthy, physically active and mentally alert.

How do these people achieve the human lifespan and avoid the common health problems that exist in our society? The answer is simple. They eat a diet high in whole grains, vegetables and fruits and low in fat, animal protein, and salt, and combine the diet with daily exercise in a pristine environment. Another interesting characteristic of these societies is respect and love for the elders, so much so that some people have been documented to exaggerate their age. It is possible for people in our society today to adopt the diet and daily exercise habits of the long-lived people described by John Robbins, but unfortunately it is impossible for most of us to find the pristine environment due to the pervasive use of chemicals in our society. Since the 1970s more than 70,000 man-made chemicals have been added to our environment without any information on the effects most of them have on human health.

In 1974 Nathan Pritikin popularized the low-fat diet and exercise lifestyle in his book *Live Longer Now.*[9] This book was followed by other books, and the Pritikin Program was featured on the nationally televised *60 Minutes* news program in 1977 as well as 1978. In 1983 John McDougall, M.D., published *The McDougall Plan*[10] and Dean Ornish, M.D., published *Stress, Diet and Your Heart,*[11] both emphasizing the value of a very-low-fat

---

[8] Robbins, John. Healthy at 100: The Scientifically Proven Secrets of the World's Healthiest and Longest-Lived Peoples. New York: Ballantine Books, 2007.
[9] Pritikin, Nathan, Jon N. Leonard, and Jack L. Hofer. Live Longer Now: The First One Hundred Years of Your Life. New York: Ace, 1974.
[10] McDougall, John, M.D., and Mary McDougall. The McDougall Plan. Nashville: Ingram Book Company, 1983.
[11] Ornish, Dean, M.D. Stress, Diet and Your Heart. New York: Henry Holt & Co, 1983.

diet. In 1998 Lance Gould, M.D., published a book, *Heal Your Heart: How You Can Prevent or Reverse Heart Disease,*[12] which also emphasized a very-low-fat diet. How does one follow this type of diet? The Pritikin daily guidelines call for 5 or more servings of complex carbohydrates (whole grains, potatoes, yams, beans, etc.), 5 or more servings of vegetables, 4 or more servings of fruit, 2 servings of nonfat dairy, and no more than 1 serving of animal protein, primarily cold-water fish or fowl, not to exceed 3½ to 4 ounces. This type of diet is low in fat (10-15 percent of calories), high in naturally-occurring fiber (35 or more grams/day), low in cholesterol (less than 100 mg/day), very low in refined sugar, and very high in naturally-occurring vitamins, minerals and antioxidants derived from whole unprocessed foods (see Figure 8.2). The diet is also low in sodium with fewer than 1.5 grams, or 1,500 milligrams per day (no added salt). In spite of the abundance of scientific evidence supporting the value of this type of diet, especially when combined with daily exercise, to prevent and/or treat many of the degenerative diseases common in our society today, most health agencies still recommend a diet with 30-35 percent of calories derived from fat. This standard was started in 1988 with the first report of dietary recommendations from the National Cholesterol Education Program[13] and has been confirmed in the third dietary recommendations released by the NCEP in 2001[14]. The present U.S. Department of Agriculture Food guidelines (MyPlate[15]) allows for 30-35 percent of calories from fat. This recommendation for a diet consisting of 30-35 percent of calories from fat persists despite the fact that numerous studies have shown that this type of diet does not stop the progression of

---

[12] Gould, K. Lance, M.D. Heal Your Heart: How You Can Prevent or Reverse Heart Disease. New Brunswick, New Jersey: Rutgers University Press, 1998.
[13] Archives of Internal Medicine, 1988; 148 (1): 36.
[14] Journal of the American Medical Association, 2001; 285 (19): 2486.
[15] http://www.choosemyplate.gov/dietary-guidelines.html

coronary heart disease, does not prevent cancer, and is not the most effective diet for the prevention or treatment of diabetes. In a study published in 2000 of 67,272 nurses followed for twelve years,[16] the investigators concluded that adherence to the dietary guidelines (30 percent fat-calorie diet) did not reduce the risk for heart disease or cancer. WHY does our government cling to a diet that has proven not to work? A diet that is not as effective as the lower-fat Pritikin-style eating plan? The answer may be that lobbying interests from extremely powerful forces, like the meat, sugar and dairy industries, may well be at work here. After all, it's tough to eat a diet high in meat and dairy and keep fat intake below 30 to 35 percent. These same lobbying interests do not seem to have influenced the World Health Organization – hence, WHO's continued support of a plant-based eating plan that is optimally 15 percent calories from fat or less.[17] That's what research has shown and that's what WHO sticks to. Finally in 2000 the American Heart Association (AHA) broke away from the NCEP dietary guidelines and simply recommended 6 or more servings of grain products per day, including whole grains, and 5 or more servings of fruits and vegetables per day with limited intake of foods high in cholesterol-raising fats (saturated and trans fats) and cholesterol.[18] These recommendations are similar to the Pritikin guidelines but unfortunately have been abandoned by the AHA and have been replaced with the USDA diet recommendations. The World Health Organization report in 2003 states:

> "Diet has been known for years to play a key role as a
> risk factor for chronic diseases. --- Traditional, largely
> plant-based diets have been replaced by high-fat,

---

[16] American Journal of Clinical Nutrition, 2000; 72 (5): 1214.
[17] World Health Organization and the Food and Agriculture Organization of the United Nations, 2003: Diet, Nutrition, and the Prevention of Chronic Diseases. Report of a Joint WHO/FAO Expert Consultation.
[18] Circulation, 2000; 102: 2284.

energy-dense [calorie-dense] diets with a substantial content of animal foods. But diet, while critical to prevention, is just one risk factor. Physical inactivity, now recognized as an increasingly important determinant of health, is the result of a progressive shift of lifestyle toward a more sedentary pattern, in developing countries as much as in industrialized ones."[19]

Clearly it is now recognized that lifestyle is a major factor responsible for much of the chronic disease seen in the world today. While these health problems have been virtually nonexistent in the underdeveloped countries, they are on the rise as these people change their diets to a Western-type diet and become more sedentary. The impact of this type of lifestyle change on the health status of people has been well documented in studies on the Japanese people living on the island of Okinawa as detailed by John Robbins in his book.

In 1975 the Japan Ministry of Health and Welfare established the Okinawa Centenarian Study that has scientifically documented that many elders have achieved the age of 100, remaining healthy and active. The ages were verified from the family registry system established in 1879 to record births, marriages and deaths. After 30 years of study, researchers reported that heart disease in the elders was minimal and breast cancer almost nonexistent.[20] Dietary analyses revealed that the elder Okinawans consumed seven servings of vegetables and seven servings of whole grains daily with two servings of soy. They also ate fish two or three times a week. The traditional diet of the elderly Okinawans is NOT a 30 percent fat-calorie diet but

---

[19] World Health Organization and the Food and Agriculture Organization of the United Nations, 2003: Diet, Nutrition, and the Prevention of Chronic Diseases. Report of a Joint WHO/FAO Expert Consultation.
[20] Journal of Gerontology, 2008; 63A (4): 338.

is in fact more like the Pritikin Eating Plan, around 10 percent fat calories with meat, poultry, and eggs making up just 3 percent of their diet; fish, about 11 percent. Unfortunately when the U.S. Armed Forces occupied the island after World War II, they introduced the Western lifestyle that included fast foods and inactivity, a lifestyle now adopted by many of the young Okinawans, and which has led to obesity and the associated chronic diseases.

Evidence Supporting a Low-Fat Diet and Exercise for Preventing or Controlling Diseases

Heart Disease

The leading cause of death in our society is cardiovascular disease (36 percent of all deaths), with heart attacks and strokes the major killers that account for 75 percent of the cardiovascular deaths. The underlying cause of most heart attacks and strokes is atherosclerosis (Chapter 2), the accumulation of cholesterol and other fatty material in the artery wall. This blockage in the arteries reduces blood flow and oxygen delivery to the heart or brain. The cholesterol that accumulates in the artery wall gets there from the blood (serum cholesterol). The higher the level of cholesterol in the blood, the more likely that it will accumulate in the artery wall.

> **In his groundbreaking Seven Countries Study in the 1950s and 60s, Ancel Keys, M.D., concluded that dietary saturated fat and cholesterol were *the* major factors leading to high cholesterol levels in the blood, and eventually, coronary artery disease.**

In his studies Dr. Keys, from the University of Minnesota, documented the relationship of serum cholesterol to coronary heart disease mortality and the impact of diet,[21] as shown in Figure 1.1. Dr. Keys measured serum cholesterol in individuals living in several cities from seven countries and correlated the cholesterol levels with coronary heart disease mortality. He then did a dietary analysis of foods eaten in the various countries and concluded that dietary saturated fat and cholesterol were the major factors contributing to the serum cholesterol levels, and eventually coronary heart disease. The country with the lowest cholesterol levels and lowest mortality from coronary heart disease was Japan. However, it should be noted that in the past 40 years since Japan has become an industrialized nation and has changed to many of our Western lifestyle habits of diet and inactivity, cholesterol levels have risen substantially and coronary heart disease is on the rise. The highest coronary artery disease (CAD) mortality was found in the lumberjacks from East Finland who consumed a very-high-fat diet (>45 percent calories). In spite of their high level of physical activity, their CAD mortality was *14 times greater* than in Japan with the very-low-fat diet and less physical activity.

One of the best examples of how lifestyle change can reduce the risk for cardiovascular deaths is the country of Finland. In 1971 one-tenth of the working-age men and women in North Karelia, Finland, were on disability due to coronary artery disease. In an attempt to rescue these young adults from the ravages of heart disease, the people petitioned the government for help. The government responded by giving them Pekka Puska, M.D., a young doctor fresh out of medical school and with a background in social science. Dr. Puska fervently believed, as did Nathan Pritikin, that heart disease was not inevitable but was lifestyle related. Dr. Puska set out to attack smoking, a diet

---

[21] Keys, A, ed. Seven Countries: A multivariate analysis of death and coronary heart disease. Cambridge, Massachusetts: Harvard University Press, 1980.

loaded with cholesterol and saturated fats, and to get inactive individuals moving. By 2000 the heart disease deaths in Finland had plunged by 75 percent.[22]

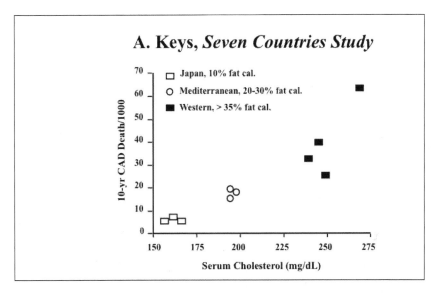

A. Keys, *Seven Countries Study*

□ Japan, 10% fat cal.

○ Mediterranean, 20-30% fat cal.

■ Western, > 35% fat cal.

Serum Cholesterol (mg/dL)

10-yr CAD Death/1000

Figure 1.1 The relationship between serum cholesterol level and coronary artery disease death rate. (Keys, A, ed. Seven Countries: A multivariate analysis of death and coronary heart disease. Cambridge, Massachusetts: Harvard University Press, 1980.)

What happens when people in the U.S. reduce the intake of dietary cholesterol and saturated fat? Figure 1.2 compares results from the Pritikin Program with published studies using the National Cholesterol Education Program (NCEP) recommendations for a 30 percent fat-calorie diet. The NCEP Step I diet allows up to 10 percent of calories from saturated fat and for Step II up to 7 percent of calories from saturated fat. Cholesterol intake is set at 300 mg/day for Step I, and 200 mg/day for Step II. It is obvious from these data on a large number of subjects that the Pritikin dietary guidelines, low in total fat (10-15 percent calories) with less than 100 mg/day of cholesterol and less than 3 percent saturated-fat calories produces

---

[22] Public Health Medicine, 2002; 4 (1): 5.

Analysis of Lipid Reductions Using
NCEP Dietary Guidelines vs Pritikin

	NCEP Step I	Step II	Pritikin
	N > 9,000		N > 4,500
Total Cholesterol	10%	13%	23%
LDL Cholesterol	12%	16%	23%
HDL Cholesterol	1.5%	7%	16%
Triglycerides	8%	8%	33%

Yu-Poth et al. Am J Clin Nutr 69:632,1999
Barnard, R.J. New Engl J Med 323:1142,1990

Figure 1.2 Serum lipid reductions with different dietary guidelines. National Cholesterol Education Program allows 30 percent fat calories while Pritikin is 10-15 percent fat calories.

a far greater drop in serum cholesterol. The reduction in serum triglycerides, another fat in the blood that contributes to coronary disease, is even more impressive on the Pritikin Program, and this is the result of not only the low-fat diet but also the daily aerobic exercise. Exercise burns fat and serum triglycerides are a readily available source of fuel that can be used by the muscles during exercise. In 1973 Dr. Oscai and coworkers reported that in men with hypertriglyceridemia (triglycerides > 200 mg/dL), 45 minutes of walking/jogging daily reduced the triglycerides down to the normal range (< 150 mg/dL) in just a few days.[23] When the men stopped exercise, the triglycerides went right back up. This emphasized the importance of daily aerobic exercise.

---

[23] Exercise and Sport Sciences Reviews, 1973; 1: 103.

> **Many studies have found that a 30 percent fat-calorie diet does *not* stop the progression of coronary heart disease. A 10 percent fat diet based on whole foods does.**

The 2003 World Health Organization (WHO) Report suggests that consuming a diet high in grains, fruits and vegetables combined with regular exercise throughout life could eradicate 80 percent of the cases of heart disease worldwide. As many developing countries move away from this type of diet and become more sedentary, the result is an increase in coronary heart disease mortality. Four studies[24] have reported a small amount of regression of coronary disease when patients are placed on a very-low-fat diet plus exercise, while many studies have reported that a 30 percent fat-calorie diet does not stop the progression of coronary heart disease. In the Stanford Coronary Risk Intervention Project[25] where regression was reported, the best predictor of new coronary blockages over the five years of observation was the dietary fat intake. As dietary fat intake rose, the number of coronary blockages rose. Those patients with the lowest intake of dietary fat (about 10 percent, like the Pritikin Eating Plan) fared the best. They had not only the lowest number of new coronary blockages but also the greatest amount of plaque shrinkage, or regression.

The benefit of dilating, or opening up, your arterial "highways"

In addition to the small amount of regression observed with the plant-based diet and exercise program is the ability of the coronary arteries to dilate or open up to increase maximum blood flow to the heart muscle. At rest, the coronary arteries are

---

[24] JAMA, 1990; 263; (12): 1646. The Lancet, 1990; 336: 129. JAMA, 1998; 280: 2001. American Journal of Cardiology, 1999; 84: 339.
[25] Circulation, 1994; 89 (3): 975.

constricted to limit the amount of coronary blood flow to the heart muscle to match the work demands of the heart determined primarily by the heart rate and blood pressure. With exercise the work of the heart increases and the coronary arteries dilate (vasodilation) to increase coronary blood flow and the delivery of oxygen and nutrients to the heart muscle. When atherosclerosis is present in the coronary arteries, it limits the amount of vasodilation that can occur and thus limits the amount of oxygen that can be delivered to the heart muscle, creating ischemia. A study was done on participants in the Pritikin Outpatient Program to measure blood flow to the heart muscle in normal subjects without coronary disease.[26] The subjects were taken to UCLA before and after the program to have blood flow to the heart muscle measured at rest and after maximum dilation with a drug. Following the 6-week program, blood flow to the heart at rest was reduced due to the reduction in heart rate and blood pressure, requiring less work by the heart. A lower blood flow at rest is good because it means your heart isn't working as hard day in and day out. These results were expected, but what was surprising was the increase in blood flow to the heart muscle following maximum drug dilation. Similar results have been reported for patients with coronary heart disease following a very-low-fat diet and exercise intervention. This improvement in the ability of the arteries to dilate is now thought to be one of the factors involved in reducing the risk for a heart attack. It makes sense. When your arterial highways are wide open, your blood cells have no problem delivering more oxygen to your heart muscle cells. Studies have also shown that one single high-protein, high-fat meal has just the opposite effect on the arteries, namely, it causes constriction (vasoconstriction) and reduces

---

[26] Circulation, 1995; 92: 197.

maximum blood flow,[27] like traffic that has slowed to nearly a standstill.

More benefits for your heart

There are many other benefits derived from a very-low-fat diet and exercise program that can reduce the risk for a heart attack. Some of the benefits include reducing risk factors such as hypertension, diabetes and obesity. There also is a reduction in inflammation and the tendency for the blood to form large clots that would block arteries already clogged from atherosclerosis. High-fat diets have also been shown to increase inflammation and to increase blood clots. This may be one of the reasons people suffer many heart attacks during the night following the typical U.S. high-fat dinner. The value of the very-low-fat diet and exercise program to reduce the risk of a heart attack and avoid bypass surgery in patients with coronary blockage has been documented. In a study[28] of 64 Pritikin Program participants with coronary heart disease and a recommendation from their physicians for bypass surgery, 81 percent had not had the bypass and only 2 had died from heart attacks 5 years after completing the program. At the start of the study, 80 percent experienced angina (chest pains) and after 5 years only 32 percent were still experiencing angina. In a similar, more recent study, 333 coronary heart disease patients who had been recommended for angioplasty or bypass surgery were given the option to attend lifestyle classes to learn about a very-low-fat diet and exercise program. Of the 333 coronary patients, 194 (58 percent) elected to try the lifestyle change as opposed to the more aggressive, expensive and risky procedures of angioplasty or bypass surgery. After 3 years, 150 (77 percent) in the lifestyle group had still

---

[27] Journal of the American College of Cardiology, 2000; 36: 1455.
[28] Journal of Cardiac Rehabilitation, 1983; 3: 183.

avoided the angioplasty or bypass, and there was no difference in events (heart attack, stroke, or death) between the two groups.[29]

Hypertension

Hypertension is defined as a blood pressure of 140/90 mmHg or higher and is a major risk factor for heart attacks, strokes and heart failure. It is the most common cardiovascular disease in the U.S. and is present in more than half of individuals, men and women, over the age of 65 years. The vast majority of people (90 percent) with high blood pressure are classified as having essential hypertension, which means that the underlying cause of the elevated blood pressure is unknown. In most of these cases, it is likely to be lifestyle related. Results of a study from the Pritikin Program show that many people with hypertension can normalize their blood pressure in 3 weeks with a low-fat, high-complex-carbohydrate, low-salt diet and daily exercise.[30] Blood pressure was reduced for the entire group (268 men and women), but more importantly 180 of the 216 patients taking medication were able to discontinue their medication while normalizing their pressure. The biggest drop in pressure was observed in the 50 patients who were not on any medication, and only 36 of the 268 patients did not respond to the diet and exercise program. Similar results were achieved in the Dietary Approaches to Stop Hypertension (DASH) study [31] conducted through the National Institutes of Health. Individuals were placed on a low-fat diet emphasizing the consumption of fruits and vegetables for 8 weeks. All blood pressure groups achieved reductions in pressures; even those with normal pressure (< 120 mmHg systolic) had a small drop. The biggest drop in pressure was observed in the individuals who were hypertensive (systolic > 140 mmHg). In another part of the study, combining salt

---

[29] American Journal of Cardiology, 1998; 82 (10B): 72T.
[30] Journal of Cardiac Rehabilitation, 1983; 3: 839.
[31] New England Journal of Medicine, 2001; 344 (1): 3.

restriction with the low-fat, fruit and vegetable diet resulted in greater drops in blood pressure. But the largest drop again was in those with hypertension, emphasizing the fact that diet is a major factor in determining blood pressure in most hypertensive patients. The 2003 report of the Joint National Committee on Prevention, Detection, Evaluation, and Treatment of High Blood Pressure[32] stressed the importance of lifestyle modification for those individuals in the pre-hypertensive range of 120 to 140 mmHg systolic. A recent study has reported that individuals in the pre-hypertensive range are at increased risk for a stroke.[33] The mechanisms for blood pressure control will be described in Chapter 3.

Diabetes

Diabetes is defined as having a fasting (no food for at least 8 hours) blood glucose (sugar) greater than 126 mg/dL or a postprandial (2 hrs. after a meal) glucose greater than 200 mg/dL. There are an estimated 24 million children and adults in the U.S. with diabetes and 6 million that are undiagnosed. Of adults in the U.S. over the age of 60 years, 23 percent are diabetic. An estimated 57 million individuals are pre-diabetic (glucose 100-125 mg/dL). There are two main categories of diabetic individuals, known as type 1 or 2. Type 1 usually develops early in life and was originally called juvenile diabetes. These individuals abruptly stop making insulin, the hormone that regulates blood glucose levels, and thus these individuals have to be on insulin injections or an insulin pump in order to live. People with type 2 diabetes, which makes up approximately 90 percent of all diabetic patients in the U.S., make some insulin but not enough, and it does not work well because they are insulin resistant. This type of diabetes is usually seen late in life and was

---

[32] http://www.nhlbi.nih.gov/guidelines/hypertension/
[33] Neurology, 2011; 77: 1330.

originally called adult-onset diabetes. However, type 2 diabetes is now being diagnosed in some children as the epidemic of childhood obesity grows.

A third type of diabetes is associated with pregnancy and is called gestational diabetes, usually associated with excessive weight gain. Although gestational diabetes may disappear after delivery, these women are at high risk for later development of type 2 diabetes.

Diabetes is the seventh leading cause of death in the U.S., but more importantly is a major risk factor for the leading cause of death -- heart disease. Individuals with diabetes are at 2-4 times the risk for heart disease compared to non-diabetics and are also at increased risk for dementia/Alzheimer's disease. The complications associated with diabetes make it a catastrophic disease. These include not only heart disease but the other atherosclerotic diseases -- cerebral and peripheral vascular disease. Diabetes is the major cause of lower limb amputations resulting from peripheral artery disease. Microvascular diseases involving the capillaries (smallest blood vessels) include retinopathy, the major cause of adult blindness, and nephropathy, the leading cause of kidney failure and renal transplants. Neuropathy involving the nerves is also commonly associated with diabetes and leads to loss of nerve function in different parts of the body.

Type 2 diabetes is a lifestyle disease with a genetic predisposition. This has been clearly demonstrated in studies conducted on the Pima Indians.[34] The Pimas who live on the Indian Reservation in Arizona have the highest incidence of type 2 diabetes of any population studied to date. Almost 50 percent of the adults develop type 2 diabetes. The high incidence of diabetes in this population has been blamed on a "thrifty gene"

---

[34] Nutrition Review, 1999; 57 (5): 55.

thought to be responsible for the high incidence of obesity and ultimately type 2 diabetes. A few years ago, a group of Pimas with the same genetic background as those from the Arizona Reservation was found living in Mexico. When they were studied, the incidence of type 2 diabetes was found to be very low, less than 10 percent. Why the difference with the same "thrifty gene" genetic background? The difference was lifestyle. Pimas living in Mexico followed the traditional lifestyle, meaning they were raising their crops, consuming far less fat and far more fruits and vegetables, and were far more physically active compared to the Arizona Pimas. These data suggest that individuals living in the industrialized countries where type 2 diabetes is common might avoid the disease if they change their lifestyle. This fact was demonstrated in the recent Diabetes Prevention Project.[35] Subjects with pre-diabetes (elevated blood glucose but not at the level defined as diabetes) were randomized into control (placebo), lifestyle change, or medication (Metformin) groups. Lifestyle change, consisting of a lower-fat diet and 150 minutes per week of brisk walking, decreased the risk for type 2 diabetes more effectively than did medication used to lower blood glucose in these pre-diabetic individuals. At 10 years of follow-up, the lifestyle intervention group still had the lowest number of subjects that had progressed to becoming diabetic.[36] It should be mentioned that the original design of the study included a fourth group on the drug troglitazone. This group was dropped as the drug was pulled from the market for adverse effects. A recent report (2011) from the National Institutes of Health suggests that up to 80 percent of all type 2 diabetes in the U.S. could be prevented by adopting a healthy

---

[35] New England Journal of Medicine, 2002; 346: 393.
[36] The Lancet, 2009; 374: 1677.

lifestyle including proper diet, regular exercise, normal body weight, not smoking and alcohol in moderation.[37]

Can Patients with Type 2 Diabetes Control their Diabetes with Diet and Exercise?

The answer is yes, especially if the lifestyle change is initiated early in the disease. The following results were obtained from the Pritikin Program. The study[38] included three groups of type 2 diabetic patients: newly diagnosed on no medication, those taking oral hypoglycemic pills and those on insulin injections. The newly diagnosed patients had the best response as glucose fell from over 160 mg/dL to 125 mg/dL in just three weeks. Only 5 of 240 patients in the group did not respond to the diet and exercise program. At the time this study was conducted, the glucose level to define diabetes was 140 mg/dL. This was recently lowered to 126 mg/dL because at 140 mg/dL many patients experience the complications of diabetes, especially coronary heart disease. The majority of patients in the Pritikin study taking oral hypoglycemic pills were able to discontinue medication and reduce their glucose while a much smaller percentage of those patients taking insulin injections were able to normalize their glucose and/or discontinue the medication. The reason for the poorer response by the patients on insulin will be detailed in Chapter 4. This is why it is important to have your glucose checked regularly and initiate the lifestyle changes immediately if your blood glucose is >100 mg/dL. A 2-3 year follow-up study of diabetic patients attending the Pritikin Program documented long-term control of diabetes through diet and exercise.[39] In addition, major lifestyle changes are likely to be more effective than the medications to reduce the risk of complications associated with diabetes, including hypertension

---

[37] Annals of Internal Medicine, 2011; 155 (5): 292.
[38] Diabetes Care, 1994; 17: 1469.
[39] Diabetes Care, 1983; 6: 268.

and the metabolic syndrome, as well as coronary heart disease. It is well documented that the majority of individuals with diabetes die prematurely from coronary heart disease. A National Cholesterol Education Program study has documented that 86 percent of diabetics have multiple risk factors (metabolic syndrome) for coronary heart disease.[40]

The Metabolic Syndrome

In 1988 Dr. Gerald Reaven from Stanford University gave the Banting Lecture at the American Diabetes Association national meeting and introduced the concept of what he called "Syndrome X," an aggregation of independent, coronary heart disease (CHD) risk factors in the same individual. The risk factors included in the syndrome were insulin resistance (hyperinsulinemia or impaired glucose tolerance), hypertension, hypertriglyceridemia, and low, high-density lipoprotein cholesterol (HDL-C). The following year Dr. Kaplan from the University of Texas called it "the deadly quartet" and Dr. Foster described it as "a secret killer." None of these acronyms described the point made by Dr. Reaven in his Banting Lecture, which was that insulin resistance/hyperinsulinemia might be the underlying cause of the syndrome. Dr. Reaven also suggested that insulin resistance and the resulting hyperinsulinemia were the underlying risk factor for type 2 diabetes, known at that time as non-insulin dependent diabetes mellitus. In 1991 Dr. E. Ferrannini, et al., published an article entitled "Hyperinsulinemia: the key feature of a cardiovascular and metabolic syndrome,"[41] terms that better reflected Dr. Reaven's point of view. Today, some individuals still use the term "insulin-resistance syndrome," but most now use the term "metabolic syndrome" (MetS) to describe the aggregation of multiple CHD and type 2 diabetes

---

[40] Diabetes, 2003; 52: 1210.

[41] Diabetologia, 1991; 34: 416.

risk factors. In addition to the factors mentioned by Dr. Reaven, Dr. Kaplan suggested that upper-body or visceral obesity needed to be considered as part of the syndrome and as a major risk factor for CHD and diabetes, independent of over-all obesity. Subsequently, many studies confirmed that abdominal obesity was correlated with the MetS[42] and its individual components. As more studies were conducted, additional CHD risk factors were added to the syndrome. Elevated serum levels of fibrinogen and tissue plasminogen activator inhibitor, both clotting factors, were related to metabolic factors for CHD as were small dense particles of low-density lipoprotein (LDL-cholesterol), all discussed in Chapter 2. The combination of elevated serum triglycerides, depressed HDL-C and small-dense LDL particles is commonly referred to as dyslipidemia and is felt to be a major risk factor for atherosclerosis.

As interest in the MetS continued to grow, several different international health agencies developed their own definitions for identifying patients with MetS, creating a lot of confusion in the medical community. In an attempt to clear up some of the controversy and unify the clinical definition of the MetS, a meeting was convened with representatives from the International Diabetes Federation Task Force on Epidemiology and Prevention; National Heart, Lung and Blood Institute; American Heart Association; World Heart Federation; International Atherosclerosis Society; and International Association for the Study of Obesity. In 2009 a "joint interim statement" was published in the journal *Circulation* establishing criteria to identify patients with the MetS.[43] There was agreement regarding the importance of central obesity; however, the cut points were different for different populations. Three abnormal

---

[42] Nature, 2006; 444 (7121): 881.
[43] Circulation, 2009; 120 (16): 1640.

findings out of five would qualify a person for MetS. The group agreed on specific cut points for triglycerides ($\geq$ 150 mg/dL or the patient is on TG-lowering meds), HDL-C ($<$ 40 mg/dL in males and $<$ 50 mg/dL in females or patients on meds), blood pressure ($\geq$ 130/85 mmHg or on meds or a history of hypertension), and fasting glucose ($\geq$ 100 mg/dL). In the U.S. the definition of abdominal obesity is a waist circumference of more than 37 inches for males and 31.5 inches for females.

As the research continued, more and more health problems have been found to be associated with the MetS and/or hyperinsulinemia. Kalmijn, et al., reported that men diagnosed with the MetS in their early 50s were more likely to develop dementia, especially vascular-related dementia, later in life.[44] In 2006 the Harvard School of Nutrition hosted a conference, *Metabolic Syndrome and the Onset of Cancer,* where several papers were presented showing that hyperinsulinemia was related to breast, prostate and colon cancers. The proceedings were published in September, 2007, in a supplement to the *American Journal of Clinical Nutrition.*[45] In a recent review, A. Galluzzo, et al., pointed out that several studies recommend that women with polycystic ovary syndrome should be evaluated for the MetS and that lifestyle modification should be the first-line therapy.[46] R. Kawamoto, et al., tested over 3,000 men and women and reported that those with the MetS had a risk ratio of 1.53 for chronic kidney disease.[47] E.A. Tsochatzis, et al., reported that insulin resistance was associated with chronic liver disease, especially hepatitis C and non-alcoholic fatty liver disease.[48] F. D'Aiuto, et al., analyzed data from 13,994 men and women from

---

[44] Arteriosclerosis, Thrombosis, and Vascular Biology, 2000; 20: 2255.
[45] American Journal of Clinical Nutrition, 2007; 86: 817S.
[46] Nutrition, Metabolism, and Cardiovascular Diseases, 2008; 18 (7): 511.
[47] Internal Medicine, 2006; 45 (9): 605.
[48] Scandinavian Journal of Gastroenterology, 2009; 44 (1): 6.

the Third National Health and Nutrition Examination Survey (NHANES) and found that individuals with severe periodontitis were 2.3 times more likely to have the MetS compared to individuals without periodontitis.[49] A.N. Vagontzas, et al., suggested that sleep apnea is also a manifestation of the MetS and is related to elevated inflammatory cytokines.[50] The mechanisms linking the MetS to CHD and type 2 diabetes are well understood, while the link to these other health problems are not well understood. D'Aiuto, et al., suggested that the chronic low-grade inflammation, characteristic of periodontitis, might contribute to the development of the MetS. Dr. W. J. Aronson of UCLA's School of Urology and I suggested that the MetS was linked to benign prostatic hyperplasia (BPH) as well as to prostate cancer risk as a result of hyperinsulinemia acting on the liver to increase production of insulin-like growth factor-I, a factor known to stimulate tumor cell growth and block tumor cell apoptosis.[51] This will be discussed in more detail in Chapter 5. It is obvious that much more research is needed before we understand how all of these factors are related from a mechanistic point of view. It is also likely that the true underlying factor is the diet (high-fat, refined-sugar) and a lack of physical activity, characteristic of the industrialized nations, and this same lifestyle being adopted in the developing countries. The metabolic syndrome will be discussed further in Chapter 4.

Cancer

Cancer is the second leading cause of death in the U.S. and had been steadily increasing until recently, when a small drop has been recorded in both the incidence and mortality of some cancers, thought to be due to early detection and better treatment, as well as more emphasis on prevention (reduced

[49] Journal of Clinical Endocrinology and Metabolism, 2008; 93 (10): 3989.
[50] Sleep Medicine Reviews, 2005; 9 (3): 211.
[51] Prostate Cancer and Prostatic Diseases, 2008; 11: 362.

smoking and discontinuation of hormone therapy in postmenopausal women). Cancer, like most of the other health problems, is primarily a lifestyle disease. The three important lifestyle factors are diet, exercise and exposure to hazardous chemicals such as cigarette smoke, pesticides, etc. These hazardous chemicals, called carcinogens, cause changes in the cellular genetic material, the DNA. Once the DNA has been damaged, the cells start to divide, forming a tumor and destroying the normal tissue where the tumor cells reside. Diet and exercise are important factors in controlling the growth of cancer cells or programming them to die. The most common solid-tumor cancers in U.S. men are prostate, lung and colon/rectal. In women the most common solid-tumor cancers are breast, lung and colon/rectal. The fat content of the diet is an important factor that stimulates cancer cells to grow. The international variation in death from prostate or breast cancers correlates with the fat content of the diet.[52] Not surprisingly, those countries with a high mortality from prostate cancer in men also have a high mortality from breast cancer in women. In addition to a difference in dietary fat intake between countries, a difference in the levels of physical activity may account for part of the large variation in prostate and breast cancer mortality observed between countries. Several large studies have shown that regular exercise reduces the risk for both of these cancers. In a study of several thousand women, participants in the National Health and Nutrition Examination Survey, women were asked to rate their consistent recreational activity level. Those women with a consistently high level of activity had a 67 percent reduction in risk for breast cancer.[53]

---

[52] Journal of the National Cancer Institute, 1998; 87: 1437. International Journal of Cancer, 1975; 15: 617.
[53] Cancer Epidemiology, Biomarkers & Prevention, 2001; 10: 805.

Several studies have investigated the relationship of physical activity to the risk of prostate cancer. In a review of 24 studies, 14 reported that occupational or leisure time activity was associated with decreased risk for prostate cancer by an average of 40 percent.[54] One study reported that 3000 kcal/week of activity reduced the risk for prostate cancer by 70 percent.[55] In the same study, conducted at the Aerobic Center in Dallas, fitness level was assessed in 12,975 men between 1971 and 1989. These men were also contacted to assess incidences of prostate cancer development for 8 years. The data showed that the higher the fitness level, the lower the risk for prostate cancer. It is also likely that the men in the highest fitness level may have had a healthier diet as they were generally more health conscious. In a recent study of 1,455 men diagnosed with localized prostate cancer, brisk walking for 3 or more hours per week was reported to inhibit or delay prostate cancer progression.[56] The mechanisms by which diet and exercise might prevent and/or aid in the treatment of cancer will be discussed in detail in Chapter 5.

Obesity

Obesity is thought to be the fastest growing health problem in the U.S. The number of obese individuals in the U.S. has increased greatly in the past 10 to 15 years. Latest statistics indicate that more than 60 percent of all adults are overweight and 30 percent are classified as being obese.[57] In addition, 15 percent of all children are severely overweight. The medical costs of overweight and obesity in the U.S. have been estimated to be more than $100 billion per year, a staggering amount.[58] The U.S. Government predicts that if the current trends continue, 42

---

[54] Cancer Causes & Control, 2001; 12 (5): 461.
[55] Medicine and Science in Sports and Exercise, 1996; 28: 97.
[56] Cancer Research, 2011; 71 (11): 3889.
[57] http://www.cdc.gov/obesity/data/adult.html
[58] Obesity Reviews, 2011; 12 (1): 50.

percent of the population will be obese by 2030.[59] Obesity is not only a problem here in the U.S. but it is now recognized as a worldwide problem. Obesity has been associated with many health problems, including type 2 diabetes, hypertension, coronary heart disease, some cancers, arthritis, gall stones and others. Unfortunately, many health professionals have indicated that obesity is the cause of these problems. While obesity may be a contributing factor, the diet one consumes and the amount of physical activity are more important. As indicated earlier, many of the problems associated with obesity, i.e., hypertension and type 2 diabetes, can be controlled in a few weeks while it takes a long time to reverse obesity.

Why are so many people becoming obese? The answer is simple but complex. In simple terms obesity can be explained by the first law of thermodynamics - energy is not created or destroyed, only transformed. This means that energy consumed in food or drink must be burned or stored. Excess energy consumed is usually stored in the body as fat. Since the 1970s energy intake per person has increased from 2,450 to 2,618 calories per day for men and from 1,542 to 1,877 calories per day for women.[60] This is due primarily to increased consumption of refined sugar. On the other side of the ledger is the fact that people are more sedentary and burning fewer calories as more time is spent watching TV, working at computers and riding in automobiles.

The increase in fat consumption is important in the development of obesity for two main reasons. First, fat has 9 calories per gram while carbohydrates and protein only have 4 calories per gram. Secondly, any excess fat calories that are consumed are easily stored while excess carbohydrate or protein

---

[59] http://www.cdc.gov/media/releases/2012/t0507_weight_nation.html
[60] http://www.npr.org/blogs/thesalt/2013/05/15/183883415/eating-much-less-salt-may-be-risky-in-an-over-salted-world

31

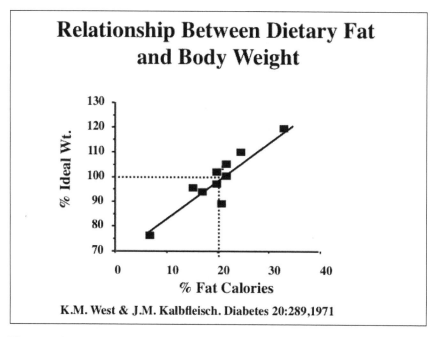

Relationship Between Dietary Fat and Body Weight

K.M. West & J.M. Kalbfleisch. Diabetes 20:289,1971

Figure 1.3 Relationship between fat consumption and ideal body weight for individual height in physically active individuals.

must be converted to fat before storage and that requires energy; in fact, almost 25 percent of the calories are burned in the conversion. Thus, it would seem that the lower the fat content of the diet, the more likely one might be able to maintain a healthy body weight. In 1970 Dr. Kelly West collected data from people in 10 different countries in Central America. He was interested in diabetes and as a part of the study he collected dietary information as well as height and weight from the subjects. Figure 1.3 is based on his data and shows that the percentage of calories from fat that was associated with an ideal body weight, based on height, was 20 percent.[61] Keep in mind that these people were far more active than most people in the U.S. today and were consuming a diet of natural foods, not all the processed

---

[61] Diabetes, 1971; 20: 289.

foods usually consumed in the U.S. today.

During the 1980s and 1990s, as American's waistlines were expanding and people were learning about fat and calories, the food industry responded by producing new low-fat or even nonfat foods. Unfortunately, many of these foods were loaded with sugar and calories even though fat content was reduced. These foods helped to contribute to the increase in fat and calorie consumption noted earlier. While dietary fat is obviously important for obesity, the amount and type of carbohydrate is also important. Simple sugars are easily absorbed into the body and cause a quick rise in both blood glucose and insulin. Insulin is known to stimulate weight gain. On the other hand, complex carbohydrates are more slowly absorbed, causing less of a rise in blood glucose and insulin. In addition, these natural foods, complex carbohydrates, that are high in water and fiber or bulk, create a feeling of fullness as opposed to processed foods full of simple sugars. A survey conducted by the U.S. Department of Agriculture on over 10,000 free-living adults revealed that those individuals with a body mass index below 25 consumed more natural carbohydrates with fewer calories, ate more grain products and fruits, and consumed less sodium. They also had the highest intake of vitamins and minerals.[62] In an analysis of data from over 120,000 health professionals, Harvard epidemiologists reported that within a 4-year period the individuals gained an average of 3.35 pounds that was strongly associated with increased daily servings of potato chips, potatoes, sugar-sweetened beverages, unprocessed red meats, and processed meats. Inverse associations with weight gain were found for the consumption of vegetables, whole grains, fruits, nuts, and yogurt.[63]

---

[62] Journal of the American College of Nutrition, 2002; 21: 268.
[63] New England Journal of Medicine, 2011; 364: 2392.

> **Recent studies have shown that the more time one spends sitting (watching TV, computer, etc.) the greater the risk for obesity and related health problems. This is true even if you have a regular exercise program.**

The importance of exercise combined with a low-fat, natural-food diet for permanent weight loss cannot be overemphasized. In the National Weight Control Registry, a study of individuals who have successfully lost weight (at least 30 lbs) and kept it off for at least one year, the average weight loss was 66 lbs. over 5.5 years. The keys for successful maintenance of weight loss were 1) a low-fat diet, 2) frequent monitoring of body weight and food intake, and 3) high level of regular physical exercise.[64] According to Dr. Hill, a co-founder of the registry, physical activity is very, very important and may be the strongest key for maintaining successful weight loss. Some have suggested that genes are a major cause of obesity. If we go back to the Pima Indian study where it has been proposed that they have a "thrifty gene," it is obvious that lifestyle is more important. In Arizona, 69 percent of Pimas who live on a high-fat diet and are sedentary are obese with a body mass index (weight corrected for height) greater than 30 while only 13 percent of the Pimas living the traditional lifestyle in Mexico, with a lower-fat diet and far more physical activity, have a BMI greater than 30.[65]

Summary

In summary, extensive scientific evidence supports the value of a very-low-fat diet with a focus on the consumption of whole grain products along with fresh fruits and vegetables to prevent and treat a majority of the diseases seen in the industrialized countries today. By its very nature, this type of diet

---

[64] American Journal of Clinical Nutrition, 2005; 82: 222S.
[65] Nutrition Review, 1999; 57 (5): 55.

is low in fat and salt while being high in fiber with an abundance of antioxidants and other needed vitamins and minerals. This type of eating pattern combined with regular exercise is nothing new but has recently been emphasized by the World Health Organization. In the WHO report, *Diet, Nutrition and the Prevention of Chronic Diseases*,[66] hundreds of scientific references are given in support of these recommendations. The fact that humans were meant to consume this type of diet is obvious from our teeth. Species that were designed to consume a high meat diet were endowed with canine teeth while humans have large, flat teeth designed for grinding grains. Another piece of physiological evidence to support the consumption of primarily a grain, legume, fruit and vegetable diet is the design of the human liver. Species endowed with canine teeth are also endowed with a liver designed to handle the high fat and cholesterol content of a high-meat diet. For example, dogs generally have cholesterol levels in the range of 60 to 80 mg/dL and do not develop coronary artery disease due primarily to the design of their livers. Humans, on the other hand, cannot cope with the fat and cholesterol contained in high-meat diets. This is obvious from the fact that at birth the cholesterol level of a human is in the same range of a dog but soon rises with consumption of the typical high-fat, high-cholesterol, refined-sugar diet.

It should also be obvious that humans, like other species, were never designed to be sedentary. This is becoming more and more obvious as our society becomes fatter and fatter. Recent studies have shown that the more time one spends sitting (watching TV, computer, etc.) the greater the risk for obesity and

---

[66] World Health Organization and the Food and Agriculture Organization of the United Nations, 2003: Diet, Nutrition, and the Prevention of Chronic Diseases. Report of a Joint WHO/FAO Expert Consultation.

related health problems. This is true even if you have a regular exercise program.[67] For many years the exercise recommendation promoted primarily by the American Heart Association was for 20 minutes of aerobic activity (walk, jog, hike, swim, cycle, etc.) three times a week. Several years ago, the American College of Sports Medicine, the premier exercise organization, recommended 30 to 45 minutes of aerobic activity 3 to 5 days a week including a warm-up and cool-down. In addition, they recommend 2 to 3 days a week of resistance or weight training to maintain muscle mass.[68] In 2002 the Institute of Medicine, U.S. National Academy of Sciences, recommended 1 hour of moderate activity daily to reduce the risk of obesity and other health problems.[69] This recommendation was confirmed in the 2003 WHO report.

The following chapters will focus on individual diseases and provide the latest scientific evidence that explains the diseases, and why diet and exercise are important preventive or controlling factors. By understanding the science and rationale for diet and exercise, individuals are more likely to be motivated to change their lifestyles. It will become clear that in some diseases diet is far more important than exercise; however, combining a diet of whole grains, fruits and vegetables with daily exercise will provide a more optimal lifestyle and improve health. It will also become clear that the underlying cause of many health problems stems from something you may have never heard of before reading this book -- free radical and inflammatory cytokine formation in the body. Although your body weight may be normal because you count calories, your body still may contain excessive amounts of free radicals and inflammatory

---

[67] American Journal of Clinical Nutrition, 2012; 95 (2) 437.

[68] Medicine & Science in Sports & Exercise, 2011; 43 (7): 1334.

[69] Institute of Medicine, Dietary Reference Intakes for Energy, Carbohydrate, Fiber, Fat, Fatty Acids, Cholesterol, Protein, and Amino Acids; September 2002.

cytokines because of the type of foods you eat, i.e., saturated fats. A diet based on whole grains, fruits and vegetables provides an abundance of antioxidants capable of combating free radicals. In addition, regular exercise enhances the body's own antioxidant mechanisms by increasing antioxidant enzymes. When Nathan Pritikin published his first book in 1974,[70] where he recommended a largely plant-based diet naturally low in fat, animal protein, refined sugar and salt, and combined with regular exercise, most of the supporting evidence was simply population relationships between lifestyle and diseases. In the past 35 years, a tremendous amount of research has provided insight into the mechanisms of how the Pritikin lifestyle might impact the common health problems seen in the industrialized nations today. The Nathan Pritikin Research Foundation lists more than 125 publications in its bibliography (Chapter 9) reporting research on the Pritikin Program including documentation of results from the Pritikin Longevity Center, studies conducted in the Metabolic Ward at UCLA, and experimental studies conducted on animals and cell cultures at UCLA.

---

[70] Pritikin, Nathan, Jon N. Leonard, and Jack L. Hofer. Live Longer Now: The First One Hundred Years of Your Life. New York: Ace, 1974.

Chapter 2

Cardiovascular Disease – The #1 Killer

Cardiovascular disease (diseases of the heart and/or blood vessels) is the number one killer in the industrialized societies of the world today and is responsible for 36 percent of deaths in the U.S. Almost 75 percent of all cardiovascular mortality in the U.S. is due to heart attacks and strokes.[71] The underlying cause of most heart attacks and strokes is atherosclerosis, the accumulation of cholesterol and other material in the artery wall that blocks the artery, reducing blood flow and oxygen delivery to the heart and/or brain. Compared to the 1960s, there has been a major reduction in cardiovascular *mortality* in the U.S. due primarily to improvements in treatment of artery disease including angioplasty, bypass surgery, and the development of drugs used for treatment. Unfortunately, there is no good evidence documenting a significant reduction in the *incidence* of cardiovascular disease; in fact, worldwide it is on the rise as the developing countries adopt a more Western lifestyle and the obesity epidemic spreads throughout the world.

The term heart disease is a general term that includes different abnormalities occurring in the heart, ranging from congenital defects that some babies are born with to the more common adult heart problems, including valve problems, arrhythmias, and coronary heart disease. Valve problems include stenosis, where the valve is scarred shut; regurgitation, where the valve does not close properly and leaks; and prolapse, where the valve turns inside out and may cause regurgitation or arrhythmia. Valve problems can lead to heart failure if not corrected.

---

[71] Circulation, 2012; 125: e2.

Arrhythmia means that the electrical activity of the heart has some defect and the various chambers of the heart are not contracting properly. Arrhythmia can be detected by feeling the pulse, with a stethoscope placed on the chest, or more precisely with an EKG recording. Some individuals take medications to control certain arrhythmias. The main arrhythmia of concern is fibrillation, where the heart muscle cells do not contract in a coordinated fashion. When this happens in the atria, the upper chambers of the heart, it has little effect on the function of the heart, as contraction of the atria is not that important for normal heart function. However, fibrillation of the atria (atrial fibrillation) can cause clots to form and collect in the lungs or go to the brain and cause a stroke. Individuals with atrial fibrillation or atrial flutter are placed on blood thinners to reduce the risk of clot formation. When fibrillation occurs in the ventricles, the lower chambers of the heart, it is a far more serious problem requiring immediate attention and defibrillation with an electric shock. If fibrillation in the ventricles is not stopped, the individuals will die as the heart stops sending blood to the brain and other parts of the body. This commonly happens to individuals when they have a heart attack.

The most common cardiovascular disease in the Westernized societies is hypertension, or high blood pressure, and will be discussed in detail in Chapter 3. Hypertension is a major risk factor for the number one vascular killer, atherosclerosis, that causes most heart attacks and strokes. Why does atherosclerosis (cholesterol deposits) develop in the arteries of so many people? The answer is simple - it is primarily lifestyles, eating habits, smoking habits, and lack of regular exercise. The first insight was gained in the very early 1900s when investigators placed rabbits on a high-fat, high-cholesterol diet. The blood or serum level of cholesterol rose dramatically, and in no time the excess cholesterol started to accumulate in the artery wall. This led to the "lipid infiltration hypothesis," which proposed that when serum levels of cholesterol exceeded physiological levels, the excess cholesterol simply filters into the artery wall and accumulates. In the 1940s pathologists studying diseased artery specimens from patients dying from heart attacks noted an infiltration of white blood cells. This observation led the pathologists to suggest that atherosclerosis was the result of inflammation in the artery wall. In the 1960s it was demonstrated in animals that injury to the delicate endothelial cells that line the artery led to the accumulation of cholesterol at the site of damage, especially if the serum level of cholesterol was high. This observation led to the "endothelial injury hypothesis" as an explanation for the development of atherosclerosis. In 1985 Drs. Brown and Goldstein from the University of Texas were awarded the Nobel Prize in Medicine or Physiology for their pioneering work with cholesterol regulation and the function of the LDL receptor. Much of their work was done using monocytes (white blood cells). They discovered that the cells would not accumulate large amounts of cholesterol unless the cholesterol was modified by chemical treatment to create oxidized or acetylated cholesterol. Antibodies were developed to detect the modified (oxidized) cholesterol, and it was soon demonstrated that oxidized cholesterol was present in the area of atherosclerosis development where the white blood cells had also accumulated in the artery wall, in both experimental animals and humans. This discovery soon led to the "lipid oxidation hypothesis" to explain the development of atherosclerosis. The combination of all of these hypotheses probably explains the development of atherosclerosis as shown in Figure 2.1. Atherosclerosis is now considered to be a disease of both excess lipids and inflammation.

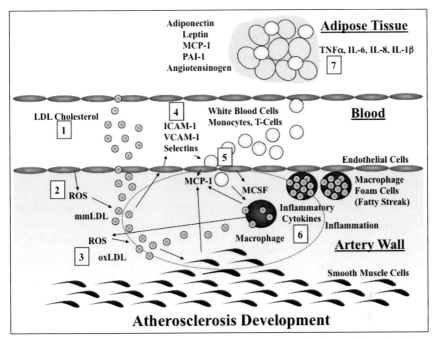

Figure 2.1 Factors involved in the development of atherosclerosis. The numbers in the boxes are thought to be the steps involved.

Atherosclerosis usually starts with an elevation of low-density lipoprotein or LDL-cholesterol in the blood (Box 1). Once the LDL-cholesterol increases above the physiological level of 80-100 mg/dL, it starts to filter into the artery wall. Inside the artery wall the LDL-cholesterol is attacked by free radicals or reactive oxygen species (ROS) initially produced by endothelial cells and later by invading monocytes (Boxes 2,3). The ROS start to oxidize the lipid content of the LDL molecule, producing minimally modified (oxidized) LDL-cholesterol (mmLDL). The mmLDL then stimulates the endothelial cells that line the inside of the artery to produce a number of chemicals known as cell adhesion molecules (CAMS) including VCAM-1, ICAM-1, Selectins, etc. (Box 4). The CAMs attract monocytes and T lymphocytes (white blood cells) in the blood to stick to the endothelial cells and enter the artery wall with the help of another molecule (MCP-1) produced by the endothelial and other cells

41

(Box 5). Once inside the artery, the monocytes are stimulated by another molecule (MCSF) that transforms them into large scavenger cells known as macrophages with scavenger receptors to take up foreign material, including oxidized LDL. This function of macrophages is normally a mechanism the body uses to protect itself from foreign invaders such as bacteria, virus, and cancer cells, and to remove cell debris. While the conversion of monocytes to macrophages is taking place, the mmLDL becomes further oxidized, including the protein component of the molecule (Box 3). This oxLDL is recognized by the scavenger receptor on the macrophages as a foreign chemical and they engulf the oxidized cholesterol molecule to hold it in the artery wall. As the macrophage fills with oxLDL, it becomes a foam cell, the hallmark of the initial stage of atherosclerosis known as a fatty streak. The macrophages also secrete ROS and inflammatory cytokines to create a state of inflammation in the artery wall that can damage endothelial cells (Box 6).

Once a fatty streak develops, atherosclerosis will usually progress to partial or complete blockage of the artery that nourishes the organ, reducing blood flow and oxygen delivery. If atherosclerosis develops in the coronary arteries that supply the heart muscle, it is called coronary heart or coronary artery disease and may eventually lead to a heart attack (myocardial infarction). If atherosclerosis develops in the carotid arteries that supply the brain with needed blood and oxygen, it is called cerebrovascular disease and may lead to a stroke (cerebral infarct). In some individuals, especially individuals with diabetes, atherosclerosis may develop in the leg arteries, known as peripheral artery disease, and may lead to claudication (leg pain or fatigue) and the possible need for amputation.

Figure 2.1 indicates the involvement of adipose or fat tissue in the development of atherosclerosis, which often involves years in the making (Box 7). Overall, obesity and especially central or abdominal obesity are well-recognized risk factors for atherosclerosis. Central obesity is a more important risk factor than over-all obesity due to the fact that abdominal fat cells generate more inflammatory cytokines than do subcutaneous fat cells. Recently, fat deposits on the heart that generally cover the coronary arteries have received attention as factors that contribute to the development of coronary atherosclerosis. Like abdominal fat cells, the myocardial fat cells release large amounts of inflammatory cytokines that could enhance atherosclerosis development and could contribute to plaque rupture, leading to a heart attack.

Although most heart attacks/strokes occur in older individuals, atherosclerosis usually develops slowly throughout life. A normal artery consists of three layers: the intima, media and adventitia (Figure 2.2). The intima, made up of one layer of

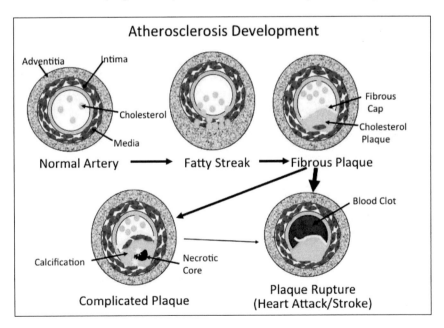

Figure 2.2 Steps in the progression of atherosclerosis leading to the heart attack or stroke.

endothelial cells, was thought for many years to simply provide a smooth surface through which the blood would flow without causing damage to the normal blood cells, and to act as a diffusion barrier to limit the amount of material, including cholesterol, that would enter the artery wall. Then in the 1980s and 90s it was discovered that the endothelial cells were capable of producing a host of chemicals that could affect blood clotting, constriction or dilation of the artery, and aid in the development of atherosclerosis. The media is the middle layer and is made up primarily of smooth muscle cells that constrict or relax (dilate) to direct blood flow to the different parts of the body. They also play a key role in determining hypertension and will be discussed in Chapter 3. The outer layer, or adventitia, is primarily a tough, connective layer that supplies support and protection to the artery.

When the blood level of cholesterol increases (LDL > 100 mg/dL), it starts to filter into the artery wall, resulting in the formation of fatty streaks by the mechanisms described in Figure 2.1. Initially, it was thought that everyone was born with normal arteries clear of atherosclerosis; however, studies done on aborted fetuses have reported that if mothers had high cholesterol, and especially if they were smokers, their fetus could already have fatty streaks – the initial stage of atherosclerosis.[72] Several studies have documented that fatty streaks are already present in the coronary arteries of teenagers in the U.S.[73] Thus, it is obvious that young people in this country need to change their lifestyles to lower their cholesterol and prevent the consequences of atherosclerosis later in life. A section on the impact of lifestyle change in young children will be included later.

In young women the onset of menstruation and associated

---

[72] Journal of Clinical Investigation, 1997; 100: 2680.
[73] Arteriosclerosis, Thrombosis, and Vascular Biology, 2000; 20 (8): 1998.

increases in estrogen provides protection by several different mechanisms and tends to arrest the atherosclerosis in the fatty streak stage until after menopause, when the atherosclerosis rapidly progresses to the next step, the fibrous plaque. Men do not have the protective effects of estrogen, and, as a result, atherosclerosis develops much earlier in life, early 20s. The fibrous plaque stage was documented in studies done on U.S. male soldiers in their 20s killed in the Korean[74] and Vietnam Wars.[75] Although the soldiers had blockages in their coronary arteries, they were not suffering heart attacks due to the fact that the coronary circulation has a dilator reserve, which means that the artery could be blocked by 40-50 percent and still deliver enough blood and oxygen to the heart muscle even at maximum exercise. This is the reason cardiac surgeons for many years did not bypass a coronary artery with less than 50 percent blockage. This was a mistake as these are the arteries that cause most heart attacks. The fibrous plaque is composed of a cholesterol mass, mostly in macrophages, covered with a fibrous cap as shown in Figure 2.2.

As cholesterol accumulates and the fibrous plaque continues to grow, Figure 2.2 shows two possible scenarios. The plaque might continue to grow, blocking more and more of the artery with a necrotic core of dead cells and calcified cholesterol covered with a thick fibrous cap. The individual may or may not experience chest pains (angina) as the heart muscle experiences ischemia (lack of oxygen) during exertion. But keep in mind: Not everyone with severe coronary blockage experiences chest pain. In almost 50 percent of heart attacks, the heart attack itself is the first chest pain. This means that people with chest pains need to pay attention to them, and, just because one does not have chest pains does not mean that he or she does not have coronary

---

[74] JAMA, 1953; 152: 1090.
[75] JAMA, 1971; 216: 1185.

artery disease. The second and more common scenario, shown in Figure 2.2, is the heart attack or stroke that occurs most of the time in an artery with less than 50 percent blockage. The plaque is lipid-rich with a thin fibrous cap that ruptures, much like a boil that ruptures, leading to the formation of a blood clot that may totally occlude, or block, the artery. The cap rupture is thought to be the result of white blood cells in the artery that are causing inflammation and activating matrix metalloproteinase-9, an enzyme that degrades the fibrous cap. Enhanced inflammation in the artery may be the result of consuming a high-fat meal, increasing ROS and inflammatory cytokine production, and may explain why most heart attacks occur at night following the typical U.S. high-fat dinner. White blood cell (monocyte) function will be discussed in detail in Chapter 6.

Once the fibrous cap ruptures and the blood clot forms, obstructing blood flow and oxygen delivery to the heart muscle, the muscle starts to die and will eventually lead to the formation of scar tissue. The formation of scar tissue, however, may be prevented if the blood clot is dissolved or removed to restore blood flow *within a few hours*. This is why it is extremely important for individuals who are experiencing chest pains to get to an emergency room *as soon as possible*. Unfortunately, many people, even those with known coronary disease, procrastinate when they experience chest pains and delay getting to the emergency room. Once the scar tissue has formed, it cannot contract and thus, the function of the muscle in that part of the heart is lost. If a lot of scar tissue forms, it may lead to heart failure, also known as congestive heart failure.

Preventing Atherosclerosis – Pritikin Results

Serum Lipids

The cholesterol and other fatty material that accumulates in the artery wall as atherosclerosis develops and advances gets there from the blood stream, and the higher the blood level of lipids, especially cholesterol, the greater the risk for atherosclerosis. When one gets a blood test, the doctor usually measures the two main blood lipids or fats, cholesterol and triglycerides, that are associated with atherosclerosis. These blood lipids, because they are fats and do not dissolve in water or plasma (the watery component of blood), are packaged as lipoproteins (lipid plus protein) to be transported throughout the body. When the doctor orders the blood test, he or she usually has the patient fast (no food) for 10-12 hours. If the blood is collected into a tube with an anticoagulant and then spun down, the lipid results are expressed as milligrams per 100 milliliters (deciliter) (mg/dL) of plasma. If the blood is allowed to clot before centrifugation, the results are expressed as mg/dL of serum. There is no major difference between the values for serum or plasma.

When the individual is told to fast, the blood results do *not* include the lipid content in the largest lipoprotein – the chylomicrons. Chylomicrons form from the fat content of the recently consumed food that has been absorbed from the intestines. The lipid content of the chylomicrons depends on the fat content of the diet. They are formed in the intestine lining and delivered to the blood stream from the lymphatic system (Figure 2.3). The primary lipid content of chylomicrons is triglyceride with some cholesterol. For many years, chylomicrons were not thought to play an important role in atherosclerosis development; however, today they are thought to be important and may play a role in heart attacks as they can enhance inflammation.

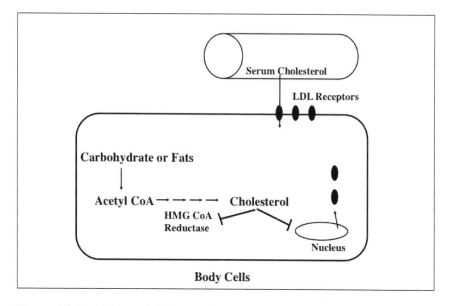

Figure 2.3 Regulation of cholesterol levels by the body cells.

As the chylomicrons circulate around the body, pieces of triglycerides are removed by muscle, especially if the individual exercises, or by fat cells where the excess calories are stored. The smaller remaining particles known as chylomicron remnants are taken up by the liver and repackaged into very-low-density lipoproteins (VLDL) that contain primarily triglyceride with some cholesterol. The VLDLs are sent back out into the circulation, and as they circulate around the body, triglyceride is again removed by muscle and fat cells, resulting in the formation of low-density lipoprotein (LDL), the primary carrier of cholesterol in the blood stream. LDL-cholesterol is known as the "bad cholesterol" as it is the cholesterol that enters the artery wall and leads to atherosclerosis (Figure 2.1).

A fourth lipoprotein is high-density lipoprotein (HDL) and is also a carrier of cholesterol. HDL-cholesterol is known as the "good cholesterol" as it is generally associated with a reduced risk for atherosclerosis. HDL proteins are formed primarily in the liver and are sent out into the circulation, where they are capable of extracting cholesterol from peripheral tissues, including the artery wall, and transporting it back to the liver where it can be degraded and excreted from the body. Think of HDL as garbage trucks. When working properly, these garbage trucks do a very good job of removing garbage (LDL "bad" cholesterol) from our arteries and transporting it to the "waste removal site" – our livers. This process is also referred to as reverse cholesterol transport. In addition to reverse cholesterol transport, HDL also contains enzymes that are antioxidants and help protect LDL-cholesterol from being oxidized, further reducing the risk for atherosclerosis. Unfortunately, there are some circumstances when HDL is unable to perform reverse cholesterol transport and becomes an oxidizing agent for LDL, thus *increasing* the risk for atherosclerosis. Exactly what causes the HDL to change its characteristics is not completely understood, but recent evidence shows that free radicals/inflammation damage the HDL and that lifestyle can be a factor, as will be discussed later.

The standard blood test, after fasting (no food for 10-12 hr.), measures total cholesterol that is contained in VLDL, LDL, and HDL. The standard test also measures the specific amount of LDL-cholesterol as well as HDL-cholesterol and the total amount of triglyceride. The National Cholesterol Education Program has specific recommendations for the various lipid levels to reduce the risk for atherosclerosis.[76] For individuals without CAD, total cholesterol should be < 200 mg/dL, LDL-cholesterol < 130 mg/dL, HDL-cholesterol > 40 mg/dL and triglycerides < 150 mg/dL. To achieve these levels, therapeutic lifestyle change, including diet and exercise, is recommended. For individuals with CAD or individuals with multiple risk factors for CAD, LDL-cholesterol < 100 mg/dL is recommended. If the recommended lipid levels cannot be achieved with lifestyle

---

[76] Third Report of the Expert Panel on Detection, Evaluation, and Treatment of High Blood Cholesterol in Adults.
http://www.nhlbi.nih.gov/guidelines/cholesterol/atp3_rpt.htm

modification, drug therapy should be added, not substituted, for lifestyle change. The Pritikin Program has always recommended a total cholesterol of 100 plus your age, not to exceed 160 mg/dL and a LDL-cholesterol < 100 mg/dL, as these levels are close to the physiological level where atherosclerosis rarely develops.

So what determines cholesterol levels in the body? It is important to realize that cholesterol is vital to the normal function of the body as it is found in cell membranes, it is a large component of nerve cells and the brain and is important for nerve signal conduction, and it is a precursor to steroid and sex hormones. Almost all cells in the body can make cholesterol from the breakdown of either carbohydrate or fats to acetyl CoA as shown in Figure 2.3 The rate of cholesterol production from acetyl CoA is determined by the action of the rate-limiting enzyme, HMG CoA reductase. Statin drugs lower cholesterol by blocking this enzyme. In addition to producing cholesterol, cells can also take up cholesterol from the blood via LDL receptors made in the cell nucleus and sent out to the cell membrane. In most cells in the body, the level of cholesterol is tightly regulated. When the level of cholesterol is sufficient to meet the cellular needs, HMG CoA reductase activity is blocked, as is the production of LDL receptors as shown in Figure 2.3. This control mechanism is important as it assures an adequate supply of cholesterol for the cells' needs without overloading the cells, as most cells have no way of getting rid of excess cholesterol.

The one organ in the body that can help to get rid of excess cholesterol is the liver as shown in Figure 2.4. The liver can break down cholesterol to bile and excrete it from the body as fecal bile. The cholesterol-lowering bile acid resin drugs work by increasing fecal excretion of bile, allowing the liver to break down more cholesterol to form bile. Dietary fiber, especially water-soluble fibers like pectin and oat bran, work by the same mechanism. The rate at which the liver can remove cholesterol from the blood is determined, primarily, by the number of LDL receptors on the liver membrane. Unfortunately, the human liver is not endowed with a large number of LDL receptors, and thus the liver has a very limited capacity to remove cholesterol from the blood to convert it to bile for excretion from the body. This is why we have to limit intake as well as production of cholesterol.

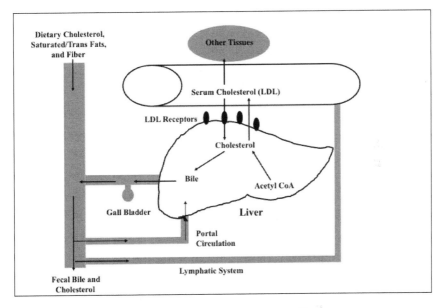

Figure 2.4. The central role the liver plays in controlling serum

There are some individuals born with genetic defects that affect cholesterol balance in the body. It has been estimated that one in every million individuals may have genetic defects and no functional LDL receptors. These individuals generally have very high blood cholesterol levels (> 1000 mg/dL) and develop atherosclerosis as very young children. One in every 500 individuals may also have genetic defects resulting in half the normal number of functioning LDL receptors and generally have blood cholesterol levels of 400-500 mg/dL and also develop atherosclerosis early in life. But for the vast majority of individuals, the impact of lifestyle, especially diet, is the major factor determining the blood cholesterol level and the risk for atherosclerosis. Table 2.1 lists the factors, mostly lifestyle, that determine serum cholesterol levels.

Factors That Determine Serum Cholesterol

Increase Cholesterol	Decrease Cholesterol
Saturated Fats	Polyunsaturated fats
Hydrogenated Oils	Monounsaturated fats
Trans Fats	Fish oil
Cholesterol	Fiber (water soluble)
Stress ?	Plant stanols
Genes	Weight loss
	Drugs

Table 2.1 Factors that affect serum (blood) cholesterol levels.

Dietary saturated fat and trans fats are the worst as they stimulate the liver to produce cholesterol and reduce the number of LDL receptors. Saturated fats are found primarily in animal products, meat and dairy, as well as in tropical nut oils including coconut and palm oil. Trans fats are manufactured fats developed to be used in margarines and baked goods. They are produced by forcing hydrogen atoms into polyunsaturated vegetable oils and are sometimes labeled as partially hydrogenated vegetable oils to make the public think they are healthy vegetable oils.

Dietary cholesterol adds to the cholesterol pool in the body. It is transported from the gut through the intestinal wall by protein carriers and is then incorporated into the chylomicrons. The number of cholesterol transport proteins in the intestinal wall determines the amount of dietary cholesterol absorbed into the body. Fortunately, most individuals only absorb about half of the dietary cholesterol they consume. Some individuals only absorb as little as ten percent of their dietary cholesterol while some, unfortunately, absorb up to ninety percent, and that greatly contributes to the serum pool of cholesterol. Factors that regulate the number of cholesterol transporters in the intestinal lining have not been investigated as the transporters have only recently been identified. Some have claimed that adding foods like eggs, high in cholesterol (egg yolks), to the U.S. diet does not raise serum cholesterol. That is like looking at a large bonfire and throwing on another log to see if the flames go higher. The important question is what happens to serum cholesterol when one removes saturated/trans fats and cholesterol from the diet. The Pritikin Program does exactly that and the data given in Chapter 1 shows that in over 4500 individuals attending the Longevity Center for three weeks, total and LDL-cholesterol were reduced by 23 percent and the vast majority of participants were able to achieve the serum cholesterol goals recommended by the NCEP.[77] Conversely when a group of Tarahumara Indians were switched from their normal low-fat, low-cholesterol, natural-food diet to a high-fat, high-cholesterol diet for five weeks, their cholesterol rose from a low of 121 mg/dL to 159 mg/dL.[78] It is important to remember that almost all dietary sources of cholesterol are also sources of saturated fat.

In addition to eliminating the dietary factors that increase cholesterol, increasing the intake of dietary factors that help to decrease cholesterol can also be important. Especially increasing the intake of water-soluble fibers and plant stanols is important. Water-soluble fibers like pectin and oat bran bind cholesterol and bile in the gut and force the body to excrete them in the feces. This allows the liver to take up more cholesterol from the blood and convert it to bile for excretion. Plant stanols are found in

---

[77] Archives of Internal Medicine, 1991; 151: 1389.
[78] New England Journal of Medicine, 1991; 325 (24): 1704.

fruits, vegetables, nuts, seeds, cereals, etc. They are molecules that have a chemical structure similar to cholesterol and can block the absorption of cholesterol from the small intestines, thus reducing blood levels of cholesterol. According to the American Heart Association, increasing the intake of polyunsaturated fats (vegetable oils) or monounsaturated fats (olive or canola oil), especially if they replace saturated or trans fats, will also reduce cholesterol. This, however, is bad advice for several reasons. Polyunsaturated fats, vegetable oils or omega-6 fats like corn oil stimulate tumor cell growth.[79] They are also precursors to inflammatory cytokines, chemicals produced in the body that incite inflammation that is associated with cancer as well as atherosclerosis, diabetes, arthritis etc., and will be discussed later in Chapter 6. Polyunsaturated fats, like other fats, are also high in calories and contribute to obesity. The answer is not to replace the fats, saturated and trans fats, but to dramatically reduce all fats except the long-chain, omega-3 fats found in cold-water fish and some nuts and seeds. This is exactly what the Pritikin Eating Plan does as it reduces fat intake to 10-15 percent of calories while increasing omega-3 fatty acid intake by including cold-water fish in the diet two to three times each week. This dramatic reduction in dietary fat intake from the typical U.S. intake of 30-40 percent of calories, along with the reduction in cholesterol, results in the 23 percent reduction in total and LDL-cholesterol reported for the Pritikin Program.

In addition to the dramatic reduction in LDL-cholesterol achieved by following the Pritikin Program, the nature of the LDL molecule is changed. It is now recognized that LDL particles in the blood exist in different sizes and densities that have different impact on the risk for atherosclerosis. Small-dense LDLs are far more atherogenic compared to large, less dense

---

[79] Carcinogenesis; 1999; 20 (12): 2209.

LDLs. The size and density of LDL is inversely related to the amount of triglyceride in the blood. Thus, it is not surprising that the Pritikin Program, reported to reduce triglycerides by 33 percent,[80] also causes a shift in the LDL molecules from small-dense to larger, less dense molecules that are known to be less atherogenic.[81]

Since triglycerides are inversely related to HDL-cholesterol in the general U.S. population, one would assume that the Pritikin Program, reported to reduce triglycerides by 33 percent, would result in a significant increase in HDL-cholesterol. In fact, just the opposite is found as HDL-cholesterol generally falls on the Pritikin Program. Some have perceived this as bad, but it may be a natural response of the body to the dramatic reduction in total and LDL-cholesterol. The high levels of triglycerides usually found in the U.S. are generally associated with a low HDL-cholesterol that is thought to increase the risk for atherosclerosis. For many years health agencies used the ratio of total cholesterol/HDL-cholesterol to calculate the risk for atherosclerosis. Data from the Framingham Heart study found that the typical ratio in the U.S., where atherosclerosis is common, was 5:1, and that a ratio less than 3.5:1 was found to be associated with low risk. More recently the American Heart Association has discontinued the use of the ratio and has focused on the absolute cholesterol values, and for good reason. Research has found that some populations with low HDL cholesterol may in fact have very low rates of heart disease. For example, the Tarahumara Indians, who live in rural Mexico, are known for a lack of atherosclerotic disease with a ratio of 5.4:1 total cholesterol/HDL-cholesterol.[82] As adults, their total cholesterol was found to be 136 mg/dL and their HDL-cholesterol 25 mg/dL.

---

[80] Archives of Internal Medicine, 1991; 151: 1389.
[81] Women's Health, 1999; 9: 155.
[82] American Journal of Clinical Nutrition, 1982; 35: 741.

Their diet was 12 percent fat calories and only 71 mg/day cholesterol, very similar to the Pritikin Eating Plan.

Like LDL-cholesterol, not all HDL molecules are identical; they vary in composition and function. Normally, HDL possesses many anti-atherogenic properties, including reverse cholesterol transport to remove cholesterol from the artery wall and deliver it back to the liver where it could be converted to bile for excretion. HDL normally contains antioxidant components that can reduce the oxidation of LDL, and it can decrease the production of cell adhesion molecules that attract white blood cells into the artery wall where they accumulate oxidized LDL to form the fatty streaks of atherosclerosis. Unfortunately, HDL does not always possess these beneficial attributes as many individuals with normal levels of HDL (> 40 mg/dL for men, > 50 mg/dL for women) still experience cardiovascular events, heart attacks or strokes. In a recent study of over 1000 individuals, the ability of their HDL to extract cholesterol from macrophages (functional capacity) was measured and was found to be a strong inverse predictor of coronary disease status.[83] In other words, the less capable a person's HDL was at extracting cholesterol (removing garbage), the more likely that person was to suffer from coronary disease.

What exactly determines whether HDL is anti- or pro-inflammatory is not known, but Navab and colleagues from the Atherosclerosis Laboratory at UCLA recently reported that pro-inflammatory HDL was found in individuals with an inflammatory response characterized by elevated C-reactive protein.[84] Elevated C-reactive protein is now recognized as a risk factor for atherosclerosis and acute myocardial infarction. As the Pritikin Program had previously been reported to reduce C-

---

[83] New England Journal of Medicine, 2011; 364: 127.
[84] Trends In Cardiovascular Medicine, 2005; 15 (4): 158.

reactive protein,[85] it was postulated that HDL might change from pro- to anti-inflammatory in response to the program and reduce the oxidation of LDL. In 22 men, all overweight/obese, and 15 with metabolic syndrome, their HDL was found to be pro-inflammatory upon entry to the Longevity Center. After 21 days at the Pritikin Center, tests showed that their total HDL was decreased, but more importantly, the HDL had converted from pro- to anti-inflammatory.[86] This functional aspect of HDL to reduce LDL oxidation may be far more important than the absolute level of HDL. The drug companies have spent considerable effort developing drugs to increase HDL in the hopes of reducing cardiovascular mortality. Unfortunately, the attempts have not met with success. In one large study with 15,000 coronary patients, the subjects were divided into one group treated with a statin and the other with the statin plus the experimental drug developed to increase HDL. The study was stopped early due to the fact that there were excess deaths (82 vs 51) in the experimental group with the elevated HDL.[87] It may be that coronary patients produce mainly dysfunctional HDL due to their lifestyle.

It is obvious from the previous discussion that the majority of individuals in the U.S. could reduce their cholesterol and achieve NCEP recommended levels through proper lifestyle modification. The few individuals unable to achieve the goals recommended by the NCEP should have drug therapy added to the lifestyle changes to reduce the risk for atherosclerosis. It is important to emphasize that the drugs should be *added* to the lifestyle changes, not replace them. Unfortunately, the NCEP or more recent U.S. Department of Agriculture dietary recommendations (USDA plate) do not allow most individuals to

---

[85] Metabolism, 2004; 53: 377.
[86] Journal of Applied Physiology, 2006; 101: 1727.
[87] New England Journal of Medicine, 2007; 357: 2109.

achieve their cholesterol goals – their recommendations are simply not rigorous enough – and many physicians ignore the lifestyle guidelines and go straight to the drugs simply because they are known to be effective for lowering cholesterol in most individuals and have been shown to reduce the risk for heart attacks and strokes in patients with atherosclerosis. In fact, many physicians never mention diet and exercise to their patients. In a study of 93 participants at the Pritikin Longevity Center (39 women, 54 men) who entered the program already taking statin drugs and having achieved a 20 percent decrease in their serum cholesterol in response to the drug, these participants achieved an additional 19 percent reduction in their cholesterol in response to the Pritikin Program.[88] In addition to the reduction in cholesterol, triglycerides fell by 29 percent. One disconcerting result from the study was the fact that 51 percent of the home physicians had used no dietary program before starting the statin drugs, and 29 percent never mentioned the importance of combining the drug therapy with a healthy lifestyle. When individuals are placed on statins by their physicians, they are told the drugs will reduce their risk for a heart attack or stroke but are not told by *how much*. A 2005 report analyzed the data from 14 randomized statin trials (5 yrs.) and found that cardiovascular events (MI, stroke, bypass) were reduced by only 21 percent, CAD mortality was reduced by 19 percent, and total mortality was non-significantly reduced by 12 percent by the statins.[89]

Oxidation of LDL

Once cholesterol filters into the artery wall, mainly due to the high concentration in the blood and/or damage to the endothelial cells that line the artery wall, the development of atherosclerosis starts with oxidation of LDL by ROS from the

---

[88] American Journal of Cardiology, 1997; 79: 1112.
[89] The Lancet, 2005; 366: 9494.

endothelial cells (see Figure 2.1). ROS, as discussed earlier, are chemically reactive molecules containing oxygen, and are also called reactive oxygen species, or free radicals. First, the outer shell of the LDL molecule is oxidized, resulting in minimally modified LDL (mmLDL, Figure 2.1). With further oxidation the protein component of LDL is also oxidized, forming oxLDL. This process of oxidation of LDL depends on the number of free radicals, mainly oxygen radicals (ROS), formed in the artery wall, and the susceptibility of LDL to be oxidized. High-fat, refined-sugar diets are known to increase the formation of ROS and increase oxidative stress and the amount of LDL that is oxidized. Switching to a low-fat, complex-carbohydrate diet reduces serum levels of markers of oxidative stress. As serum usually contains several antioxidants (i.e. vitamins), capable of reducing ROS, the measure of serum levels of markers of oxidative stress may not reflect the amount of ROS present in the artery wall formed by the endothelial cells and macrophages once they accumulate. In order to investigate the impact of lifestyle on the formation of ROS by endothelial cells, and in doing so, possibly reflect what is going on in the artery wall, we cultured human artery endothelial cells and stimulated them with serum obtained from participants at the Pritikin Program. Compared to the samples obtained upon entry into the program, the post-program samples showed a significant reduction in ROS formation.[90]

Many individuals in the U.S. take antioxidant vitamin supplements (i.e., vitamins C, E, beta-carotene, etc.) hoping to reduce their risk for cancer and heart disease. Unfortunately, many trials have shown no benefit from taking supplements to prevent either cancer or heart disease. In fact, taking vitamin E

---

[90] Journal of Applied Physiology, 2006; 100: 1657.

supplements increased lung cancer in smokers.[91] In CAD patients taking statin drugs, vitamin E supplements had an adverse effect on serum lipids.[92] On the converse, numerous studies have reported that individuals who obtained their antioxidants by consuming large amounts of fruits, vegetables and whole grains reduced their risk for both cancer and heart disease. Most people do not consume the minimum number of five serving of fruits and vegetables daily recommended by the U.S. Department of Agriculture, and most people are unaware of the value of natural foods. As the old saying goes, " An apple a day keeps the doctor away." One single red apple has the antioxidant equivalent of 1500 mg of vitamin C supplement. In addition the apple contains pectin, a water-soluble fiber that helps reduce cholesterol.

Another factor that determines the amount of oxidized cholesterol that accumulates in the artery wall is the susceptibility of LDL to oxidation. This depends on the size and density of the LDL molecules as well as the amount of antioxidants incorporated in them, including vitamin E and beta-carotene. Both of these factors can be altered by proper diet and exercise. Using serum samples obtained from participants in the Pritikin Program, we isolated LDL for testing. When we measured the size and density of the LDL in the pre-program samples, most of the LDL was small and dense. In the post-program samples, the LDL was predominately large, less dense.[93] When we measured the vitamin E and beta-carotene content of the LDL, we found the beta-carotene content to be significantly increased (46 percent) in the post samples. The amount of oxidized LDL in the serum was

---

[91] American Journal of Respiratory and Critical Care Medicine, 2008; 177: 524.
[92] JAMA, 2005; 293: 1338.
[93] Arteriosclerosis, Thrombosis, and Vascular Biology, 1996; 16: 201.

significantly reduced in the post samples compared to the pre-program samples. The isolated LDL was then subjected to oxidation with copper sulfate, a common oxidizing agent. In the post-program samples the LDL was far more resistant to oxidation: the rate of oxidation was reduced as was the maximum amount of oxidation. Thus, not only does the Pritikin Program dramatically reduce the total amount of LDL-cholesterol in the blood that is available to enter the artery wall, it also alters the LDL molecules to make them more resistant to oxidation -- a key factor in the accumulation of cholesterol in the artery wall.

Recruiting Monocytes into the Artery Wall

Once the LDL-cholesterol enters the artery wall and the cholesterol oxidation process starts, the mmLDL is recognized as a foreign chemical and the artery responds by stimulating the production of a number of factors by the endothelial and smooth muscle cells that recruit white blood cells (monocytes, T-lymphocytes) into the artery wall. The first factors stimulated to increase are cell adhesion molecules (CAMs) including ICAM-1, VCAM-1, selectins, etc. These CAMs move into the endothelial cell wall where they attract the white blood cells floating in the blood stream to stick to the endothelial cells. The white blood cells are then transported into the artery wall by monocyte chemotactic protein-1. Some of the CAMs inserted into the endothelial cell wall will be released into the blood, where they can be measured. In serum samples obtained from Pritikin Program participants, lower levels of CAMs were found in the serum after the diet and exercise intervention. Endothelial cells were then grown in cultures and stimulated with the Pritikin serum. The post-program serum resulted in a lower level of CAMs being produced and fewer white blood cells sticking to the endothelial cells.[94] Collectively, these data indicate a reduction in the risk for atherosclerosis development.

Inflammation in the Artery Wall

Figure 2.1 shows that in the area in the artery where atherosclerosis develops, inflammatory factors, including cytokines released from the macrophages and fat cells, and C-reactive protein (CRP) accumulate. As discussed earlier, C-reactive protein is a marker for inflammation and is recognized as a risk factor for atherosclerosis and myocardial infarction. CRP is released into the blood stream when there is a general infection in the body, and the levels of CRP increase up to 100 to 1,000 mg/L. It is the chronic, lower levels of CRP indicative of chronic low-grade inflammation that are of concern and are referred to as hs-CRP (high-sensitivity CRP) as it takes a special assay to measure the very low levels. According the American Heart Association hs-CRP lower than 1.0 mg/L is low risk for atherosclerosis, 1-3 mg/L is average risk, and higher than 3.0 is high risk. A value higher than 10 mg/L indicates systemic infection, and the test needs to be repeated at a later date after the infection is treated. In men attending the Pritikin Program, hs-CRP was reduced from 2.4 ± 0.5 to 1.5 ± 0.3 mg/L,[95] in women it was reduced from 2.6 ± 0.5 to 1.4 ± 0.2 mg/L[96] while in overweight/obese children it was reduced from 3.61 ± 0.7 to 2.14 ± 0.05 mg/L.[97] Other markers of inflammation, including serum amyloid A, IL-6, IL-8, and TNFα were also reduced in serum from Pritikin Program participants.[98] The level of localized inflammation in the atherosclerotic lesion is important as

---

[94] Journal of Applied Physiology, 2006; 100: 1657.
[95] Journal of Applied Physiology, 2006; 100: 1657.
[96] Metabolism, 2004; 53: 377.
[97] Atherosclerosis, 2007; 191: 98.
[98] American Journal of Physiology: Endocrinology & Metabolism, 2012; 303: E542.

increased inflammation is thought to be a factor activating the enzymes matrix metalloproteinases (MMPs) that leads to plaque rupture and myocardial infarction. In men attending the Pritikin Program one of the MMPs, serum MMP-9, was reduced from 779 ± 85 to 626 ± 61 ng/mL, indicating a reduction in the risk for an acute myocardial infarction.[99]

Risk Factors

In addition to cholesterol, especially LDL-cholesterol, other risk factors identified in epidemiological studies like the Framingham Heart Study that are associated with the development of atherosclerosis include hypertension, diabetes, and the metabolic syndrome. Being diabetic has the same risk for a heart attack as does having documented coronary disease. All three of these risk factors respond very well to the Pritikin Program and will be discussed in separate chapters. In addition, physical inactivity is recognized as an important risk factor and is one of the reasons that regular exercise is an important part of the Pritikin Program.

Treating Atherosclerotic Patients – Pritikin Results

Coronary Artery Disease

When Nathan Pritikin wrote his first book in 1974, he stated that the Pritikin Program could reverse atherosclerosis and eliminate the need for bypass surgery. Unfortunately, he had no scientific data to support his claims other than the fact that he felt he had reversed his own heart disease. In 1958, during a comprehensive medical examination, he was diagnosed with ischemic heart disease based on a stress test showing ischemic changes in the electrocardiogram (EKG). His cholesterol was 280 mg/dL, and that is when he developed the Pritikin Program. After a few years of following his diet and doing daily walking, his

---

[99] Journal of Applied Physiology, 2006; 100: 1657.

cholesterol had dropped to a low of 102 mg/dL, and the results of additional stress tests revealed no ischemic EKG changes. He also cited animal studies showing that exercise might stimulate the development of collateral vessels around the blockage in the coronary arteries, and thus he thought that daily exercise was important. The autopsy conducted following his death in 1985 revealed: "No elevated plaques were present, and no reduction in the lumen [inner open space of the arteries] was found."[100]

Scientific evidence to support Mr. Pritikin's claim that his program could eliminate the need for bypass surgery came in 1983 with the publication of a 5-year follow-up study of 64 coronary heart disease patients who had attended the Pritikin Longevity Center.[101] All 64 patients had been recommended for bypass surgery by their personal physicians based on coronary angiograms documenting blockage in one or more of their coronary arteries. However, the patients elected to forgo the surgery and attend the Pritikin Program. At 5 years of follow-up, 52 of the patients (81 percent) still had not had the bypass. Before entering the Pritikin Program, 80 percent of the patients experienced angina. At follow-up, only 32 percent indicated they definitely had angina. At 5 years after having been recommended for bypass and having attended the Pritikin Center, only four patients had died -- two from coronary events, one from cancer and one during surgery for a heart valve replacement -- for a total mortality of only 6 percent. This very low mortality rate can be compared with the Veterans Administration Bypass Surgery Study[102] of high-risk patients where the 5-year mortality rate was 38 percent for the group randomized to standard medical care and 17 percent for those who had the bypass. Some of the Pritikin patients who were diagnosed with coronary disease in their 50s or

---

[100] New England Journal of Medicine, 1985; 313: 52.
[101] Journal of Cardiac Rehabilitation, 1983; 3: 183.
[102] New England Journal of Medicine, 1984; 311 (21): 1339.

60s made it to their 80s and 90s without ever having the bypass. For example, Danny, an insurance executive had been a track athlete at Michigan State University in the 1930s but gave up exercising after college as he spent 10 hours-plus daily working. Then, at age 64, he suffered a heart attack. He was recommended for bypass surgery but instead went through the Pritikin Longevity Center's 26-day program. His cholesterol dropped from 285 mg/dL to 147 mg/dL and his weight dropped from 176 to 159 pounds. Danny also discontinued all of his heart medications. Twenty-two years later, he was still visiting the Longevity Center for his biannual visit, just as a refresher. He never had another heart problem. Four days a week, this octogenarian was jogging three miles, and twice weekly he lifted weights with a personal trainer. And at age 86, Danny was still working three days a week at his insurance office.

The presence of angina is commonly used as an indicator for more aggressive treatment of coronary disease, i.e., angioplasty or bypass surgery. Thus, the fact that the Pritikin Program participants lost their angina supports the lack of need for bypass by using appropriate lifestyle intervention. In a more recent publication, Frattaroli, et al., (2008) reported on a much larger study in which 158 coronary patients experienced activity-limiting angina and 90 patients had mild angina. After 12 weeks of lifestyle intervention, including a 10 percent fat-calorie diet and moderate exercise, 186 of the patients were angina-free and 23 reduced their angina from limiting to mild.[103] There were 24 patients who were angina-free at entry into the study but developed signs of angina at 12 weeks. A more recent study has confirmed the Pritikin Program results documenting the fact that coronary patients can avoid bypass surgery with appropriate lifestyle change. From a group of 333 coronary patients, all

---

[103] American Journal of Cardiology, 2008; 101 (7): 911.

recommended for coronary revascularization, 194 elected to try lifestyle change in place of the more aggressive and risky procedures (angioplasty/bypass) and were compared with 139 patients who had the procedures. After three years, there was *no* difference between the two groups for myocardial infarction, stroke, non-cardiac or cardiac deaths.[104]

So why do coronary patients undergoing aggressive lifestyle change do so well? Do they actually regress their coronary disease as Mr. Pritikin postulated, or are there other factors that reduce their risk for myocardial infarction? As stated in Chapter 1, four studies have documented a small amount of regression in coronary blockage with aggressive lifestyle changes including diet and exercise, while patients on standard medical care (30 percent fat-calorie diet and appropriate drugs) showed increased blockage. These results suggest that other factors are also important. The study by Czernin, et al.,[105] on Pritikin Program participants, without coronary disease, showing an increase in the ability of the coronary circulation to vasodilate (open up) and increase maximum coronary blood flow may be an important factor and has recently been confirmed in a study on exercise training in coronary patients by Hambrecht, et al.[106] The increase in the ability of the coronary vessels to vasodilate was associated with an increase in nitric oxide synthase, the enzyme involved in the production of nitric oxide, a powerful vasodilator (to be discussed at length in Chapter 3 on hypertension). In patients with documented CHD, Gould, et al.,[107] studied myocardial perfusion (the amount of blood flowing to the heart muscle) by PET in 20 patients who were directed to follow a 10 percent fat-calorie diet, mild-to-moderate exercise, and stress

---

[104] American Journal of Cardiology, 1998; 82: 72T.
[105] Circulation, 1995; 92: 197.
[106] Circulation, 2003; 107 (25): 3152.
[107] Journal of the American College of Cardiology, 2003; 41: 263.

management intervention, and in 15 control patients with standard medical care including the NCEP 30 percent fat-calorie diet. From baseline to 5 yrs., there was improvement in maximum blood flow to the heart in the intervention group, while the blood flow was reduced in the control group. In a subsequent study, this same group studied the effects of combined lifestyle and statin therapy on myocardial perfusion by PET over a 2.7 yr treatment span. They had three treatment groups of coronary patients, designated as "Poor" (no statin or lifestyle treatment), "Moderate" (statin alone or statin plus the NCEP diet or a 10 percent fat-calorie diet alone), and Maximal (statin plus a 10 percent fat-calorie diet and exercise). Over the period of observation, perfusion decreased in the Poor group, stabilized in the Moderate, and improved in the Maximal treatment group. At 5 yrs follow-up, only seven percent in the Maximal group experienced any coronary-related event compared to twenty percent in the Moderate group and thirty-one percent in the Poor group.

Other factors that might be involved in the reduction in risk for myocardial infarction resulting from intensive lifestyle change include stabilization of the cholesterol plaque resulting from reduced inflammation, and a reduction in the risk for blood clot formation. As discussed earlier, most heart attacks occur as a result of plaque rupture in arteries blocked less than 50 percent. Once the plaque ruptures, the plaque material is exposed to the blood and results in the aggregation of blood platelets that stimulate the blood clot to form and block the artery. Many coronary patients take aspirin to reduce platelet aggregation and the tendency for the blood to clot. Studies on Pritikin Program participants have shown a reduction in the tendency for platelets to aggregate[108] and clots to form. Rupture occurs in what is

---

[108] Prostaglandins, Leukotrienes and Medicine, 1987; 26: 241.

known as vulnerable plaques -- cholesterol-rich plaques with a high level of inflammation. The inflammation is thought to activate enzymes like matrix metalloproteinases that degrade the fibrous cap covering the cholesterol plaque, making it vulnerable to cracking or rupture. As discussed earlier, the Pritikin Program has been shown to reduce markers of inflammation as well as the level of one of the metalloproteinases (MMP-9), which should immediately reduce the risk for plaque rupture, clot formation and a heart attack.

Peripheral Artery Disease (PAD)

The development of atherosclerosis in the large arteries in the legs is called peripheral artery disease. Although PAD is usually not a life-threatening condition, it can be very debilitating and can lead to the need for amputation when gangrene develops in the feet due to a lack of blood supply. Patients with PAD can be severely limited in their exercise capacity due to claudication pain or simply extreme fatigue in the legs with exercise. The condition was initially called peripheral vascular disease or PVD.

The development of atherosclerosis in the legs is no different than the development of atherosclerosis in the coronary arteries; the same mechanisms are thought to be involved. Because it is the same disease in two different places, the same dietary advice is given to reduce lipids and other factors associated with atherosclerosis. What *is* different is the exercise prescription given to the patients. Patients with coronary artery disease are assigned a level of exercise based on their heart rate response during a graded exercise test and/or signs of ischemia (EKG changes/angina). The training or exercise heart rate is set at the heart rate just below the rate where ischemic changes are noted in the electrocardiogram during an exercise stress test or at the level where angina develops. It is important that the patient does not exceed the assigned heart rate to avoid the development of ischemia and the risk for a heart attack. Conversely, the leg muscles have a high capacity for anaerobic (without oxygen) metabolism and cannot be damaged (as heart muscle can) by exercising to the point of ischemia. Thus, PAD patients are told to walk to the point of severe leg pain, sit down and rest, and, when the pain subsides, get up and walk again to the point of severe pain. This process is repeated until the patient has walked for 45-60 minutes. At least two exercise sessions are recommended each day. The rationale for exercising to the point of severe pain is to make the leg as ischemic as possible to stimulate the formation of collateral vessels around the blockage to improve blood flow to the lower leg.

Using this exercise prescription combined with the Pritikin diet has been shown to be highly effective for dramatically improving performance capacity in PAD patients in just a few weeks. In a study of 16 PAD patients attending the Pritikin Program, it was reported that the patients had improved blood flow to the legs and increased their walking, that was minimal before the program, to over 2 hours each day at the end of the program.[109] The improvement in blood flow to the legs was associated with the elimination of claudication pain in 11 of the 16 patients during the PVD Doppler test as well as a 61 percent increase in maximum work capacity during a progressive treadmill test. In a case report of one PVD patient,[110] the improvement in performance was quite dramatic and was associated with the documented development of collateral vessels. A 46-year old male, pre-Pritikin, suffered with severe claudication pain upon walking. He had no palatable pulses at his ankles, indicating severe PAD. An arteriogram was performed that revealed 100 percent occlusion (complete blockage) of both femoral arteries at mid-thigh with some reconstitution of flow by

[109] Journal of Cardiac Rehabilitation, 1982; 2: 569.
[110] Physician and Sports Medicine, 1982; 10: 90.

small collaterals just below the knee. The man was recommended for immediate bypass surgery. He had read Nathan Pritikin's book *Live Longer Now* and decided to try the Pritikin Program in place of the surgery. When he arrived at the Pritikin Longevity Center, he could walk no more than 100 yards before the pain in both legs forced him to stop. Following the Pritikin exercise prescription for PAD patients, he noticed immediate improvement, and by the end of three weeks he was able to walk 3 miles in one hour with minimal leg pain. Upon returning home, he continued to follow the Pritikin diet and to walk, and then started to add jogging. His performance improved to the point that he ran several 10K races with minimal pain as long as he did not go too fast. In a little over a year after leaving the Pritikin Center, he completed the Chicago Marathon. When Nathan Pritikin heard of the patient's miraculous feat, he was convinced that the man had regressed the blockage in his legs. It was explained to Mr. Pritikin that regression was unlikely as the vessels below the blockage were not visible on the arteriogram and had likely disappeared. What was more likely was the development of a massive collateral network of vessels around the blocked area. Mr. Pritikin contacted the man and invited him back to the Pritikin Center for additional testing. The patient was found to have good pulses at the ankles at rest and a Doppler test showed blood flow at all levels of both legs, although the flow signal was abnormal especially in the right leg. An exercise Doppler test was administered that showed a normal response in the left leg but an abnormal response in the right leg. The patient was taken to the University of California, Irvine, Medical Center where a digital arteriogram was performed. The results showed that a massive collateral network of vessels had developed, and especially in the left leg the deep femoral artery had dilated to enhance blood flow. Other studies discussed in the publication have also reported improvements in performance with exercise in

PAD patients, but nothing as dramatic as this case. This was the first documentation of the development of collateral vessels in a PAD patient resulting from an intensive exercise program. The ability of some PAD patients, with less than complete occlusion of femoral arteries, to regress their atherosclerosis was reported by Brandt, et al., using a low-fat diet and cholesterol-lowering drugs.[111]

Collectively, these data indicate that the Pritikin Program for diet and exercise, when combined with appropriate medical management, should be highly effective for both the prevention and treatment of atherosclerotic diseases. As heart attacks and strokes resulting from atherosclerosis are responsible for more deaths than any other single factor and are responsible for a tremendous amount of the shockingly high medical costs reported annually in the United States, adopting the Pritikin Program should be a priority of any responsible citizen.

Reducing Atherosclerosis Risk in Children

As indicated earlier, several studies have documented the presence of fatty streaks in the arteries of teenagers growing up in the U.S. The extent of atherosclerosis in the coronary arteries of young boys correlated with the extent of obesity. This observation indicates that the present epidemic of obesity in children will result in an increase in coronary heart disease in future adults, and there is an urgent need to change the lifestyles of young people. In the summer of 2002, the Pritikin Longevity Center instituted a special family program where adults could bring their children for a two-week program. Everyone was placed on the Pritikin diet, and special lectures and exercise classes were offered to the children. The exercise involved 2 to 2.5 hours of supervised exercise daily including gym-based workouts in the morning and a variety of activities in the

---

[111] Annals of Internal Medicine, 1977; 86: 139.

afternoon, including tennis, beach games, swimming, etc. Data were initially obtained from 19 overweight subjects ranging in age from 8 to 17 years.[112] During the 2-week session the children lost an average of 8.8 pounds but were still diagnosed as being in the overweight range when they returned home. Despite still being overweight at the end of the program, the children achieved dramatic reductions in factors associated with atherosclerosis. Changes in serum lipids are shown in Table 2.2

In addition to the major reduction in serum lipids, other serum factors associated with atherosclerosis development were reduced, including markers of oxidative stress (8-isoPGF$_{2\alpha}$ and myeloperoxidase) and soluble cell adhesion molecules (ICAM-1, E-selectin). Serum levels of C-reactive protein, an inflammatory marker, were reduced from 3.6 to 2.1 mg/L, and MMP-9 was reduced from 1484 to 761 ng/mL, indicating reduced inflammation. When the serum was used to stimulate endothelial cells grown in culture, the cells produced fewer oxygen radicals (ROS) while increasing the production of nitric oxide in the post-program compared to the pre-program serum. The increase in nitric oxide production agrees with the reduction in blood pressure (130/74 to 117/67 mmHg) observed in the children. Serum insulin, a risk factor for atherosclerosis and the metabolic syndrome, was reduced from 27.2 to 18.3 µU/mL in response to the intervention. If these children continue to follow the Pritikin Program at home, they should continue to lose weight and dramatically reduce their risk of developing atherosclerotic disease as adults.

---

[112] Atherosclerosis, 2007; 191: 98.

Effect of the Pritikin Program on Children's Lipids, N=19

	Pre	Post	% Decrease
Total Cholesterol (mg/dL)	158±8	125±6	21
LDL-Cholesterol (mg/dL)	89±8	67±6	25
HDL-Cholesterol (mg/dL)	42±2	43±3	---
Total-C/HDL-C	3.9±0.3	3.2±0.3	19
Triglycerides (mg/dL)	134±15	82±8	39

Table 2.2 Lipid changes in children attending the Pritikin Program for 2 weeks.

In a more recent paper with data from 33 children,[113] 19 overweight/obese and 14 lean, who had attended the Pritikin Longevity Center it was reported that not only did overweight/obese children reduce their heart disease risk factors so did the normal weight children. These data indicate that body weight per se may not be a good indicator of heart disease risk in children.

---

[113] *Am J Physiol Regul Integ Comp Physiol.* In Press 2013.

Chapter 3

Hypertension (high blood pressure)

As stated in Chapter 1, hypertension is usually defined as a blood pressure equal to or higher than 140/90 mm Hg and is the most common cardiovascular disease in the U.S. For individuals with diabetes or kidney disease, a value of 130/80 mmHg is used. Although hypertension has been known for many years to be a major risk factor for heart attacks, strokes, and heart failure, recent data show that even pre-hypertension (>120/80,<140/90) is a significant risk factor for strokes. Pressure is usually measured in a large artery (brachial) in the upper arm. A cuff with a sphygmomanometer to measure pressure in the cuff is placed around the arm and inflated until no sound can be heard with the stethoscope placed over the artery below the cuff. The cuff is slowly deflated until a sound in the stethoscope detects blood flowing. This is when the pressure in the cuff is equal to the pressure in the artery and is recorded as the systolic pressure or the pressure when the heart is contracting and ejecting out blood. The cuff is further deflated until no sound is heard and this pressure is recorded as the diastolic pressure or the residual pressure in the artery when the heart is relaxing and filling with blood. Hypertension can be due to either a rise in the systolic or the diastolic pressure, or in many cases both pressures are elevated.

The important questions are, what causes blood pressure to rise from a normal value of less than 120/80 mm Hg, and what role does lifestyle play in the rise in pressure? Let's look first at factors that might cause blood pressure to rise. There could be an increase in the amount of blood pumped out of the heart, known as the cardiac output. This is what happens when you exercise.

The heart pumps out more blood and the pressure rises. Second, there could be an increase in resistance to blood flow that is caused by constriction (vasoconstriction) in arteries, especially the small arteries (arterioles), or hardening or calcification of large arteries. Thirdly, rising blood pressure could be due to an increase in blood or plasma volume, exerting excess pressure on the artery walls. Limited evidence suggests that individuals with hypertension might have a cardiac output at rest that is a little greater than that of normotensive individuals, but it is not thought to be a major cause of hypertension. That leaves us with the other two factors, and there is good evidence to show that both, increased resistance and plasma volume, play significant roles in most of the hypertension seen in people in the U.S.

Vasoconstriction/Plasma Volume

Constriction or dilation of blood vessels is important for the regulation and distribution of blood flow throughout the body. This regulation is extremely important during exercise as some arterioles are constricted to reduce blood flow to the liver and kidneys, while others are dilated to increase blood flow to the heart and skeletal muscles. For the detection of hypertension, blood pressure is measured at rest when blood flow is low. At rest, a balance between factors that cause arterioles to constrict or dilate determines the resistance to blood flow and consequently the blood pressure. As discussed in Chapter 2, the medial (middle) portion of the artery wall is comprised primarily of a layer of smooth muscle cells. It is the constriction or dilation of these smooth muscle cells that primarily determines the resistance to blood flow and ultimately pressure in the arteries. Figure 3.1 indicates that there are three main factors that determine the state of contraction or relaxation of the smooth muscle layer in the arteries: nitric oxide (NO) (Box 1), sympathetic nerve innervation (Box 2), and angiotension II, a protein in the blood (Box 3).

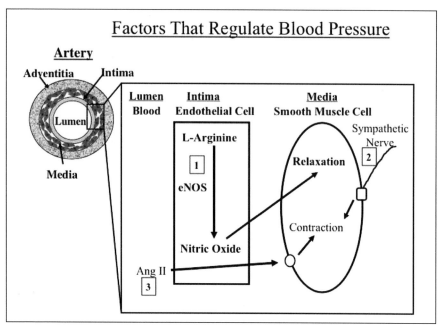

Figure 3.1 Three factors that constrict or dilate arteries.

NO (Box 1 in Figure 3.1) is a powerful smooth muscle relaxer (vasodilator) discovered in the body in the 1980s and shown to cause vasodilation of the arteries. Vasodilation is simply a scientific term for dilation – the widening of the "inner pipeline" (lumen) of blood vessels. NO is produced from the amino acid L-arginine obtained from dietary protein. Its production is regulated by the activity of the enzyme nitric oxide synthase (eNOS). Once NO is produced by the endothelial cells, it diffuses into the smooth cells and causes relaxation. Think of it as our own naturally-derived muscle relaxer. NO is a gas and only lasts for a few seconds. Thus, it has to be continually produced to cause vasodilation of the arteries. When an eNOS blocker is given to reduce NO production, the result is a rise in blood pressure to the hypertensive level. This indicates that to have a normal blood pressure the arteries must continually produce NO. Shear stress created by the velocity of blood flowing over the endothelial cells, like the stress that exercise creates, stimulates eNOS, resulting in increased NO production. This is why regular exercise is so important for maintaining normal blood pressure. A second physiological factor that stimulates eNOS is estrogen, which explains why women, prior to menopause, generally have much lower blood pressure than men.

The sympathetic nervous system (Box 2 in Figure 3.1) sends nerves from the cardiovascular center in the brain stem to innervate the artery's smooth muscle cells (and kidneys). These nerves activate alpha-adrenergic receptors that subsequently cause the smooth muscle cells to contract (vasoconstriction). When an individual with normal blood pressure is given an alpha-adrenergic blocker to reduce sympathetic nervous system activity, the blood pressure shows a small drop. This indicates that at rest there is some sympathetic vasoconstriction; however, it is much less than the NO-induced vasodilation.

The third factor that regulates vasoconstriction, and also regulates plasma or blood volume (the amount of blood flowing through our blood vessels), is angiotensin, part of the renin-angiotensin-aldosterone system (RAAS) shown in Figure 3.2 (Box 3 in Figure 3.1). The RAAS was designed to compensate for an unexpected blood loss resulting in an abnormal drop in blood pressure. This was part of our evolutionary heritage developed to compensate for a loss of blood from predators like saber-toothed tigers and other humans. When there is an unexpected blood loss, blood pressure drops and the sympathetic nervous system is activated. The increased sympathetic nervous system activity signals the kidneys to release a hormone called renin into the blood stream. Renin acts on a protein angiotensinogen, released from the liver and fat cells, and

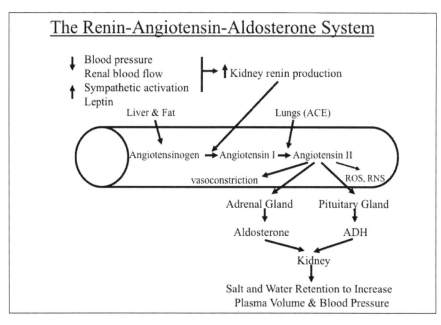

Figure 3.2 The renin-angiotensin-aldosterone system and how it affects blood pressure.

converts it to angiotensin I, a relative inactive protein. As angiotensin I passes through the lungs, it is acted on by an angiotensin converting enzyme (ACE) that converts it to angiotensin II. Angiotensin II also acts on the adrenal and pituitary glands to release hormones (aldosterone and antidiuretic hormone) that in turn act on the kidneys so they retain salt and water to increase plasma volume. This is obviously an important mechanism the body uses when blood pressure drops from excessive blood loss, but unfortunately, over activity of the system without a blood loss results in elevated pressure and can cause hypertension. Over activity of the RAAS and excessive production of angiotensin II could be caused by increased sympathetic nerve activity resulting from hyperinsulinemia, causing blood pressure to rise.

Another factor that can activate the RAAS is the protein leptin released into the blood stream from fat cells. Plasma leptin levels are directly correlated with the level of body fat, and thus provide a mechanism explaining the well-documented relationship between obesity and hypertension. Exactly how leptin increases RAAS activation is not known, but the good news is that serum levels of leptin can be substantially reduced with just a few weeks of proper diet and exercise, long before obesity is controlled, and will be discussed later in Chapter 6. Over activity of the RAAS must play an important role in the development of hypertension as many drugs used to treat hypertension work on the RAAS. For many years the most common drugs used to treat hypertension were diuretics that reduced plasma volume. Newer drugs include ACE inhibitors and ARBs (angiotensin receptor blockers) that directly reduce RAAS actions and lower blood pressure. ACE inhibitors block the conversion of angiotensin I to the active angiotension II while the ARBs block the action of angionsin II at its receptor.

What Causes Hypertension and What Role Does Lifestyle Play?

Endothelial Dysfunction

Numerous studies in humans using flow mediated dilation (FMD) measurements have reported defects in endothelial function (inability of the endothelium to produce sufficient NO). FMD tests are conducted by placing a pressure cuff around the upper arm just as when we measure blood pressure, inflating the cuff to restrict blood flow to the arm for a period of time, and then deflating the cuff rapidly to measure blood flow below the cuff using a Doppler flow probe. As discussed earlier, one of the important factors that stimulates or activates eNOS to increase NO production and vasodilation is shear stress. FMD tests are thus measuring the ability of shear stress created by rapidly deflating the cuff to stimulate NO and increase blood flow as a measure of endothelial function. As numerous studies have documented endothelial dysfunction in hypertensive patients, we must ask: What causes the endothelial dysfunction and what role does lifestyle play?

In an attempt to answer these two questions, we conducted a series of animal studies. When young rodents were placed on a high-fat, refined-carbohydrate/sugar diet (HFS) where 40 percent of the calories were obtained from fat (lard, saturated and monounsaturated fats) and 40 percent from refined sugar (sucrose), similar to the typical U.S. diet loaded with refined carbohydrates (white flour bread, pretzels, bagels, white rice, white pasta), blood pressure increased.[114] In male rats on the high-fat, refined-sugar diet, blood pressure started to increase after 2 months and reached the hypertensive level by 4.5 months. In rats fed a low-fat, complex carbohydrate diet (LFCC), blood pressure remained normal. In female rats, blood pressure in the HFS group was elevated at 6 months but did not reach the hypertensive level until 2 years, when the rats were in menopause. This is the exact situation that is observed in humans. Males in the U.S. start to develop hypertension in their early 20s while females generally don't develop hypertension until after menopause. These observations indicate that estrogen is an important factor in blood pressure regulation. It is well known that estrogen activates eNOS and increases the amount of eNOS in endothelial cells to increase NO production. We went one step further and obtained ovariectomized, young female rats and placed them on the HFS diet. At 7 months the ovariectomized female rats were hypertensive just like the males on the HFS diet.[115] When estrogen was replaced with estrogen pellets, blood

---

[114] Roberts, C.K., A. Izadpanah, S. Angadi, R.J. Barnard. Effects of an intensive short-term diet and exercise intervention: Comparison between normal weight and obese children. *Am J Physiol Regul Integr Comp Physiol.* In press 2013.

[115] Journal of Applied Physiology, 2001; 91: 2005.

pressure was normalized in one month in the young ovariectomized females on the HFS diet.

These studies clearly demonstrate that the typical high-fat, refined-carbohydrate diet leads to hypertension. The good news was that in both male and postmenopausal female rats with HFS-diet-induced hypertension, blood pressure was normalized by switching the rats from the HFS to the LFCC diet for 2 months. Was the HFS diet-induced hypertension a result of endothelial dysfunction? To answer this question we conducted several studies. First, we gave the postmenopausal rats a drug to block the eNOS for 2 days. In the LFCC rats the drug caused blood pressure to elevate to the hypertensive range while in the hypertensive HFS rats there was only a small, further increase in blood pressure.[116] These results were interpreted as indicating a defect in eNOS function in the hypertensive HFS rats and showed that in the rats on the LFCC diet with normal blood pressure, nitric oxide was causing a significant amount of vasodilation. The rats were then placed in metabolic cages for two days to collect urine and measure nitric oxide metabolites. In the hypertensive HFS rats, NO metabolites were barely detectable while the LFCC rats with normal blood pressure excreted large amounts of NO metabolites.[117]

To further document that the HFS diet-induced hypertension was the result of endothelial dysfunction and a lack of NO vasodilation, artery strips were isolated from both diet groups and studied in chambers to test for NO-induced vasodilation. The artery strips were contracted and given various doses of a drug to stimulate eNOS to cause vasodilation. The artery strips from the hypertensive HFS animals showed only half the relaxation observed in the LFCC group. Again, when the

---

[116] Hypertension, 2000; 36: 423.
[117] Hypertension, 2000; 36: 423.

animals were switched from the HFS diet back to a LFCC diet for one month, blood pressure was normalized. When the artery strips were studied in the chamber using the drug to stimulate eNOS, the response in the switch-back group had normalized to the level observed in the LFCC group. After a brief recovery period the artery strips were again contracted and treated with another drug to directly stimulate the smooth muscle cells to relax (vasodilate). The response in all three groups was normal, showing that the abnormal relaxation response in the HFS group was isolated to defects in the endothelial cells in the artery lining.[118] Figure 3.3 summarizes the effects of diet on artery vasodilation and blood pressure.

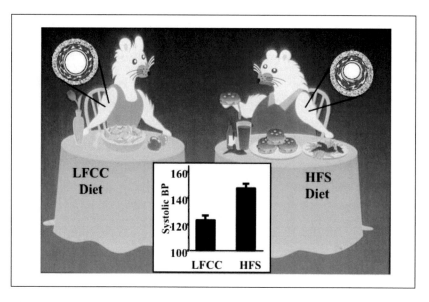

Figure 3.3 Effects of diet in rodents on artery function and blood pressure.

So what was causing the endothelial defect and the observed lack of NO vasodilation in the HFS group? We hypothesized that the HFS diet decreased the amount of eNOS in

[118] Surgical Research, 1999; 85: 96.

the endothelial cells resulting in a reduction in NO production. We also hypothesized that NO produced in the endothelial cells in the HFS animals were being inactivated by reactive oxygen radicals (ROS). Both of these hypotheses turned out to be correct. eNOS protein content in the arteries of the HFS animals was found to be half that of the LFCC arteries. Serum markers of oxidative stress and ROS formation were substantially elevated in the HFS animals, and the nitrogen radical content of the arteries was increased by at least fifty percent, indicating inactivation of NO.

Increased Sympathetic Nervous System Activity

Indirect evidence, including increased resting heart rate and elevated levels of plasma and urinary catecholamines (sympathetic neurotransmitters) commonly found in hypertensive patients, supports the concept that hypertension is due, at least in part, to increased sympathetic nervous system activity, causing vasoconstriction and activating the RAAS. These indirect measures did not permit scientists to conclude that sympathetic overdrive was a major factor in most cases of hypertension. More recently the development of sophisticated techniques have allowed a more direct assessment of sympathetic function. The direct measurement of peripheral sympathetic nerve firing has provided conclusive information documenting enhanced sympathetic activation in hypertensive as well as in pre-hypertensive individuals. In addition, recent tests show that the increased peripheral sympathetic activity is associated with enhanced central sympathetic activity in the brain.[119]

So what causes the increased sympathetic activity? Some have suggested that hormonal factors, including angiotensin II, leptin, and/or insulin, may be the underlying cause either through central or peripheral mechanisms. Blood levels of these

---

[119] Hypertension, 2009; 54: 690.

hormones are usually all elevated in hypertensive patients and are commonly associated with obesity. Insulin infusions into animals and humans have been shown to increase sympathetic activity. Hyperinsulinemia as a result of insulin resistance is commonly found in patients with metabolic syndrome and/or type 2 diabetes, as well as hypertension, and will be discussed in Chapter 4.

Increased Plasma Volume

In view of the well-documented increase in sympathetic activity and vasoconstriction in peripheral tissues, including the kidney, it is not surprising that the RAAS would be activated and play a significant role in hypertension. When the arterioles in the kidney are constricted, blood flow to the kidneys is reduced, and that activates the RAAS. Elevated plasma levels of angiotensin II and aldosterone are well documented in hypertensive patients. In addition, the Framingham Offspring Study (which is tracking more than 5,000 men and women who are the children of the original subjects of the renowned Framingham Heart Study) reported that rising levels of aldosterone in normotensive subjects predicted subsequent development of hypertension.[120] There is an old saying in kidney physiology: "As salt goes so goes water." This means that if the kidneys retain salt they also retain water, and plasma volume increases and can contribute to hypertension. Increased levels of both aldosterone and ADH, resulting from activation of RAAS, force the kidneys to retain salt and water.

This brings us back to an old friend NOS, responsible for producing NO. It is located not only in endothelial cells of the artery lining as depicted in Figure 3.1, but also in kidney epithelial cells. Studies on isolated kidney preparations have shown that NO production forces the kidney to excrete sodium, and that means that water will follow to reduce plasma volume.

---

[120] Circulation, 2011; 124: e466.

In our studies described previously on rats made hypertensive by placing them on a high-fat, refined–carbohydrate/sugar diet, we found that the diet not only reduced NOS and NO in the artery, the same response was observed in the kidneys. It's interesting to note that these results were achieved on a low-salt diet, which shows that fat and refined carbs, not just excess salt, play a key role in inducing hypertension. When the hypertensive HFS animals were placed on a high-salt diet, their blood pressure rose *even higher*, suggesting kidney dysfunction and the inability of the kidneys to excrete the excess sodium. The Pritikin Eating Plan is very low in sodium and thus the body is less likely to accumulate excess fluid resulting in increased plasma volume.

Collectively, these data indicate that the underlying causes of most hypertension involve endothelial dysfunction (lack of NO production and vasodilation), sympathetic vasoconstriction, and activation of RAAS to increase plasma volume and also cause vasoconstriction. All of these factors can be induced by a high-fat, refined-carbohydrate/sugar diet with excess salt like that commonly consumed by individuals in the U.S., where hypertension is so very common.

As people are living longer, we are seeing older individuals with isolated systolic hypertension and low diastolic pressure. This is associated with hardening/calcification of large arteries, mainly the aorta. Normally, when the heart contracts and ejects blood out into the aorta, the elastic components stretch to accept the blood and then recoil during diastole to keep the blood moving throughout the body as the heart fills with blood for the next beat. When the aorta becomes hard due to calcification, it cannot stretch and causes systolic pressure to increase. This forces more blood down the arteries during systole and results in a low diastolic pressure because there is no recoil in the aorta. Exactly what causes the hardening/calcification of the aorta is unknown. Also it is unknown if lifestyle change can prevent or reduce the hardening/calcification of the arteries.

Treatment of Hypertension with Lifestyle Change – Can It Be Effective?

In Chapter 1, two studies were described documenting that lifestyle change can lower blood pressure. The DASH study using only a low-fat diet with an emphasis on consuming fruits and vegetables high in antioxidants, showed that after eight weeks, blood pressure was reduced, even in the group with normal blood pressure -- less than 120/80 mm Hg.[121] When salt restriction was added to the diet, a further reduction in blood pressure was noted, especially in the hypertensive group. The second study was done on hypertensive patients attending the Pritikin Longevity Center, where the low-fat, low-salt, high-complex-carbohydrate diet was combined with daily exercise. Many of the patients were taking drugs to control their blood pressure when they entered the program, and they still had a drop in pressure, and many were able to discontinue their drugs.[122] To date, seven papers from the Pritikin Program have been published that included data on hypertensive patients. Roberts and Barnard combined the data from all seven studies that are shown in Figure 3.4. In this large population of patients with hypertension (N=1117), blood pressure was reduced close to the normal levels. More importantly, a little more than half of the 598 patients initially taking antihypertensive medicine were able to stop taking their drugs.[123] So what is it about the Pritikin Program of diet and exercise that might prevent or treat hypertension?

[121] New England Journal of Medicine, 2001; 344 (1): 3.
[122] Journal of Cardiac Rehabilitation, 1983; 3: 839.
[123] Journal of Applied Physiology, 2005; 98: 3.

Both components of the program are important for many reasons. First, let's look at the diet. It is low in sodium, less than 1500 mg per day (< 4 g of salt). This low sodium intake is

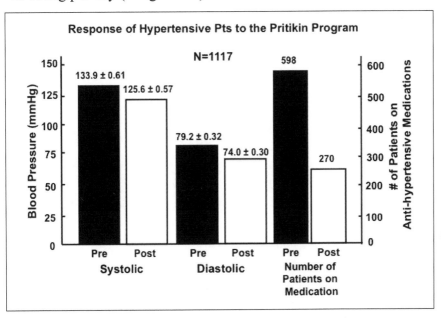

Figure 3.4 Response of hypertensive patients to the Pritikin 3-week diet and exercise program. Data from Roberts and Barnard *Journal of Applied Physiology,* **2005; 98: 3.**

achieved by avoiding all processed foods where salt is commonly used as a preservative and flavor enhancer, and not adding salt to the natural foods that make up the Pritikin Eating Plan. The relationship between salt consumption, a rise in blood pressure with adult aging (20-59 yrs), and the development of hypertension was established by the Intersalt study[124] conducted in the 1980s. This was an international study that involved over 10,000 subjects from 52 centers in 32 countries around the world. The subjects from most centers showed an increase in blood pressure with increasing age that was correlated with salt intake; the greater the salt intake, the greater the percentage of subjects

[124] Hypertension, 1989; 14: 570.

with hypertension. In four remote populations where salt intake ranged from 1-3g (about 400 to 1,200 mg of sodium) per day or less, there was a slight or no rise in pressure with aging, and hypertension was almost nonexistent. Many individuals in the U.S. consume 8-10 or more grams of salt (about 3,200 to 4,000 mg of sodium) daily. In 1997 Dr. Stamler wrote that the INTERSALT study results are in agreement with findings from clinical observations, therapeutic interventions, randomized control trials, as well as animal studies that support the value of salt reduction for reducing blood pressure and other cardiovascular diseases.[125] One of the more impressive studies documenting the value of salt restriction was recently published by Dr. Pimenta, et al., on a group of drug-resistant, hypertensive patients. The patients were taking an average of 3.4 different drugs daily and had blood pressures of 146/84 mm Hg. In a randomized cross-over design with a washout period between a high-salt or low-salt diet, both systolic and diastolic pressures fell by 22.7 and 9.1 mm Hg, respectively, going from the high-salt to the low-salt diet.[126] These data demonstrate the importance of dietary salt reduction for treating hypertension, especially in drug-resistant patients. The link between salt intake, hypertension and cardiovascular disease is so convincing that some health groups have suggested that the government should pass legislation restricting salt content of processed foods. In support of this concept Dr. Bibbins-Domingo et al., published a paper in the *New England Journal of Medicine* entitled "Projected Effect of Dietary Salt Reductions on Future Cardiovascular Disease." They concluded that a population-wide reduction of dietary salt of up to 3 g/day (1200 mg of sodium) might reduce the annual number of new cases of coronary heart disease by 60,000 to 120,000, stroke by 32,000 to 66,000, and myocardial infarction

[125] American Journal of Clinical Nutrition, 1997; 65 (suppl): 626S.
[126] Hypertension, 2009; 54: 475.

by 54,000 to 99,000, and reduce the annual number of deaths from any cause by 44,000 to 92,000. These reductions were estimated to save $10 to $24 billion annually – all this money saved simply from reducing salt intake by 3 g/day.[127] In the INTERSALT study of remote populations, where hypertension was rare and correlated with a very-low-salt intake, the individuals also had a low-fat, high-fiber diet of natural foods high in potassium, which is thought to counteract some of the effects of high sodium intake.[128] Most of these people were also very active physically. All of these factors are important for preventing/controlling hypertension. That's why they are all incorporated into the Pritikin Program.

As discussed previously, our rodent experiments demonstrated that a high-fat, refined-carbohydrate/sugar diet, similar to the typical U.S. diet, resulted in hypertension associated with endothelial dysfunction, increased oxidative stress, reduced nitric oxide production, and reduced endothelial NOS content. As the Pritikin Program has been shown to be effective in controlling hypertension, usually by replacing the typical high-fat, refined-carbohydrate/sugar diet with the Pritikin low-fat, complex-carbohydrate diet, correcting these factors must be contributing to lowering blood pressure. Several studies have reported significant reductions in markers of oxidative stress in Pritikin Program participants, as discussed in Chapter 2, on the involvement of oxidative stress in atherosclerosis development. In a study of 11 men who attended the Pritikin Program (7 with hypertension), we reported a reduction in both systolic (19 mm Hg) and diastolic (8 mm Hg) pressures along with a 30 percent reduction in 8-iso-PGF$_{2\alpha}$, a marker for oxidative stress.[129] The men were asked to collect 24-hour urine samples to measure

[127] New England Journal of Medicine, 2010; 362: 590.
[128] Hypertension, 1989; 14: 570.
[129] Circulation, 2002; 106: 2530.

nitric oxide metabolites. The results showed a 30 percent increase in NO metabolites in the post-program samples indicating increased NO production. This increase in NO metabolite excretion could be due to less scavenging of NO by free radicals (ROS) or could be due to increased production of NO. In all likelihood both factors are involved in the increase in NO metabolites. The reduction in serum 8-iso-PGF$_{2\alpha}$ would suggest less scavenging by oxygen radicals. A number of studies have reported that adding an array of fruits and vegetables to the diet, as found in the Pritikin Eating Plan, reduces oxidative stress associated with an increase in beneficial phytochemicals with increased serum oxygen radical-absorbing capacity. In addition, the daily exercise would increase shear stress to activate eNOS and increase NO production, resulting in vasodilation to reduce blood pressure. Many studies have shown that regular exercise training improves flow-mediated vasodilation in humans, and studies in rodents have reported that training increases eNOS protein content of arteries. Training has also been reported to increase antioxidant enzymes in the body that would add to the oxygen-radical absorbing capacity.

Does the Pritikin Program reduce sympathetic nervous system vasoconstriction of arteries? Although not measured directly, the answer would seem to be yes based on the fact that two of the factors thought to stimulate the cardiovascular centers in the brain stem to increase sympathetic vasoconstriction, leptin and insulin, are both reduced by the Pritikin Program. Both of these factors are also associated with obesity. Fasting insulin was reduced in response to the Pritikin Program in three studies with adults and one study with children. In the children's study, leptin was recently measured and was reduced in the post-program serum by more than 50 percent, despite the fact that the children, though they had in fact lost a little weight between the pre-Pritikin testing and post-Pritikin testing two weeks later, remained overweight or obese.[130] In addition to the reduction in these two serum factors, the Pritikin Program has been reported to lower resting heart rate suggesting a decrease in sympathetic nervous activity.[131] It is well known that trained individuals have lower heart rates and blood pressures at rest and at any submaximal workload. This may, in part, be due to the ability of exercise to reduce insulin and will be discussed at length in Chapter 4. If sympathetic nervous system vasoconstriction of arteries is reduced by the Pritikin Program, one would assume a reduced activation of the RAAS. This, in combination with the increase in NO in the kidneys, would increase sodium excretion and lead to a reduction in plasma volume, placing less stress on the artery wall.

Thus, it appears as though the Pritikin Program evokes several different mechanisms to lower blood pressure and control hypertension without the need for drugs. These include increased NO availability to cause vasodilation, decreased sympathetic nervous system activation to reduce vasoconstriction of vessels, and increased ability to excrete sodium to reduce RAAS activation and plasma volume as well as reducing sodium intake.

Erectile Dysfunction

Erectile dysfunction (ED) is defined as the inability to get and/or sustain an erection. The exact incidence of ED is unknown but it is commonly found with aging and the associated health problems (heart disease, diabetes, periodontitis, and hypertension) observed in men in the U.S. ED is four times more common in men in their 60s compared to men in their 40s. Erection begins with sexual stimulation either tactile or mental. Sexual arousal causes nerves from the brain running to the penis

---

[130] American Journal of Physiology: Endocrinology and Metabolism, 2012; 303 (4): e542.
[131] Metabolism, 2006; 55: 871.

to be activated and release nitric oxide. The released nitric oxide dilates blood vessels resulting in an increased blood flow into the penis, causing an erection. A lack of nitric oxide production and/or function results in ED. Two common drugs used to treat ED, Viagra and Cialis, work by increasing available nitric oxide. Thus, the previous discussion regarding the impact of diet and exercise on nitric oxide suggests that the Pritikin Program should help to reduce the risk for ED.

Chapter 4

Diabetes and the Metabolic Syndrome

As explained in Chapter 1, diabetes is defined as having a fasting blood glucose ≥126 mg/dL or a postprandial (following a meal or glucose load test) glucose ≥200 mg/dL. Normal fasting blood glucose is 80-100 mg/dL, and the difference between normal and diabetic is referred to as pre-diabetic. So what determines the level of blood glucose? Under normal fed conditions, glucose contained in carbohydrate foods is released by digestive enzymes in the mouth and intestines, and the glucose enters the portal circulation and passes through the liver where some is stored as glycogen, as shown in Figure 4.1. Under fasting conditions or while consuming a very-low-carbohydrate diet, the body breaks down the stored glycogen to release glucose into the circulation. This is important to maintain an adequate level of blood glucose for the brain as glucose is the primary metabolite for the brain. Once the stored glycogen is depleted, the liver starts to break down protein and converts it into glucose.

The rate at which dietary carbohydrates are digested and the glucose released to enter the portal circulation depends on the nature of the foods and how fast the enzymes can digest them. Common sugar (sucrose) consists of a glucose molecule connected to a fructose molecule. Sugar can be readily digested to release the glucose molecule to enter the circulation.

Many processed foods are loaded with sugar, especially low-fat or nonfat processed foods. Other processed foods that contain refined carbohydrates, i.e., white breads, white rice and pasta, are also readily digested and quickly release glucose for absorption into the circulation. These simple sugar and/or processed foods lead to a rapid rise in blood sugar (glucose) and should be avoided, especially for individuals with diabetes. Complex carbohydrates, i.e., fruits, vegetables and whole grains high in fiber (starchy foods), are slowly digested due to their chemical nature and the presence of fiber. Since they are slowly digested, they slowly release glucose and have less of an effect on blood insulin and glucose. The fibers that make up the complex carbohydrates are not digested, slow down the digestion of other carbohydrates, and pass down the intestines into the feces taking cholesterol and water with them. These are the main foods that make up the Pritikin Eating Plan and are especially important for individuals with diabetes.

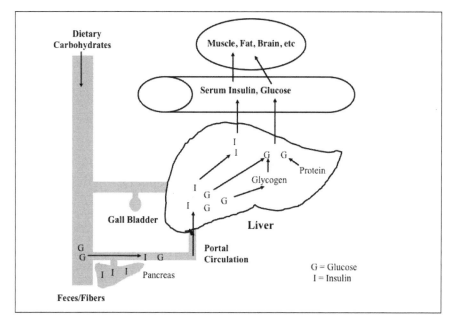

Figure 4.1 Insulin (I) and glucose (G) regulation in the body.

Once the dietary carbohydrates are digested and the released glucose enters the portal circulation, it passes by the pancreas where the concentration of glucose is sensed. In response to the glucose concentration, the beta cells in the pancreas release insulin that enters the circulation and along with the glucose passes through the liver into the general circulation for delivery to the body cells, especially the muscles and brain where it is used for fuel, or to the fat cells to store excess calories as shown in Figure 4.1. Insulin plays a key role in the entry of glucose into the body cells and will be explained shortly.

What Causes Diabetes?

Type 1 diabetes (previously known as juvenile onset or insulin dependent diabetes) is an autoimmune disease in which the immune system's white blood cells fail to recognize the pancreatic cells as part of the normal body and attack and destroy them. Why this happens in certain individuals is not exactly known. It is known that type 1 diabetes tends to run in families, suggesting a genetic link, and a few genes, especially ones linked to the immune system, have been identified. Ironically, the onset of type 1 diabetes often occurs immediately following an event like a virus attack that activates the immune system. Although the disease runs in families, studies on identical twins with the same genes show that both twins get the disease in only 50 percent of the time, indicating an important lifestyle component. Type 1 diabetes can develop in children, teens or even in adults, especially women as late as the 40s.

Onset of type 1 diabetes is accompanied by symptoms, including increased thirst, increased urination, and rapid weight loss due to the body's inability to transport glucose from the blood into the cells, due to the lack of insulin. Blood levels of glucose may reach 200-300 mg/dL, and glucose can be detected in the urine. Once insulin therapy is started, blood glucose levels fall, and, due to the fact that not all of the pancreatic cells are initially destroyed, the individual may experience a "honeymoon" phase where little injected insulin is required for a period of time with normal blood glucose levels. The duration of the honeymoon phase varies, and scientists are still trying to figure out the best way to extend the honeymoon phase. Eventually the individual will require more insulin as the honeymoon phase comes to an end and the pancreas stops making insulin. The keys for longevity free from complications (macro- and micro-vascular disease) for a type 1 diabetic are a consistent lifestyle including a healthy diet, like the Pritikin Eating Plan, daily exercise, and constant blood glucose measurements to regulate insulin for good glucose control.

Type 2 diabetes, previously known as adult-onset diabetes, is generally observed in older individuals; however, today it is being diagnosed at younger ages, even in some children. It was also known as Non-Insulin-Dependent Diabetes Mellitus (NIDDM) primarily due to the fact that most patients initially are not insulin deficient but actually have elevated levels of insulin. The problem is that the insulin is not effectively working to transport glucose from the blood into the body cells; the individuals are insulin resistant. Like type 1 diabetes, there is clear evidence for a genetic basis for type 2. Studies done on identical twins show that in 80-90 percent of the cases both twins end up with the disease. Although there is a genetic basis for the disease, the studies conducted on the Pima Indians described in Chapter 1 clearly demonstrate that lifestyle is a more important factor determining whether or not the disease develops. Figure 4.2 shows the progression of the disease that usually takes place over many years of eating the typical U.S. high-fat, refined-sugar diet, along with a lack of regular exercise. Individuals with a healthy diet and regular exercise generally have fasting insulin levels ranging from 5-10 $\mu U/mL$, and their glucose is in the normal range of 80-100 mg/dL. As lifestyle starts to change, as individuals become less active and gain weight, their muscle and liver cells become resistant to the action of insulin. Blood levels of glucose start to rise as the liver releases glucose, and uptake by muscle, the most important tissue in the body for insulin action, becomes insulin resistant. As the muscles and liver become more and more insulin resistant, glucose rises to the pre-diabetic stage (100-125 mg/dL), and the pancreas responds by releasing more insulin. This progression to the pre-diabetic stage is usually, but not always, associated with excess weight gain.

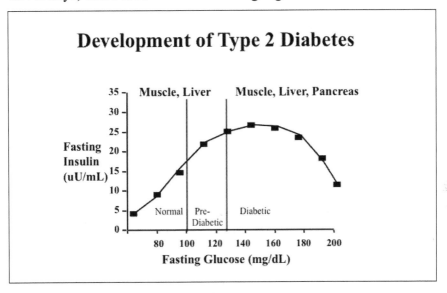

Figure 4.2 Blood glucose and insulin levels leading to type 2 diabetes.

Eventually glucose rises to the diabetic level (≥ 126 mg/dL) with severe insulin resistance. As the glucose continues to rise, insulin levels drop as the pancreas "wears out" and reduces the insulin output, resulting in the patient taking insulin. The drop in insulin release from the pancreas is now known to be due to a reduction in the number of beta cells where insulin is produced. The beta cell mass may start to decline in individuals with pre-diabetes, which means the existing cells have to work harder to produce more insulin.

Recent studies with cultures of pancreatic cells, with animal models, and with tissues obtained from diabetic patients have started to shed light on the underlying defects that cause the decline in beta cell mass and insulin levels observed in type 2 diabetes. Pancreatic tissue obtained from type 2 patients at autopsy have shown not only reduced beta cell mass but also infiltration of inflammatory white blood cells, elevated levels of inflammatory cytokines, and the accumulation of amyloid deposits, all known to induce beta cell death. The cell culture studies as well as the animal models point to the role diet can play in increasing inflammation in the pancreatic beta cells. Both glucose and saturated fatty acids have been shown to activate the inflammatory pathways in beta cells to increase inflammatory cytokines, leading to apoptosis or death of the beta cells. Regulating inflammation will be discussed in detail in Chapter 6.

Amylin is a protein hormone produced and released from the beta cells of the pancreas, along with insulin, in response to dietary sugar and saturated fat ingestion. In high concentration amylin also causes cell death of beta cells. As insulin resistance forces the pancreas to produce more and more insulin, it also produces and releases more amylin. The increased amylin production is thought to result in the formation of amyloid deposits in the pancreas. Recent studies with beta-cell cultures have found that, unlike insulin production that responds primarily to exposure to dietary glucose, amylin production is also increased upon exposure to saturated fatty acids,[132] indicating that diet is a significant factor in determining beta cell death. Cell culture studies have also shown that the inflammatory cytokine TNFα that is increased in obesity can increase amylin production. TNFα associated with diet-induced obesity will be discussed in Chapter 6. Whether it is a high concentration of amylin in the pancreatic beta cells or the formation of the amylin aggregates (plaques) that leads to destruction of the beta cells is still being investigated. Obviously, treating insulin resistance

---

[132] American Journal of Physiology: Endocrinology and Metabolism, 2010; 298: E99.

with appropriate lifestyle changes to reduce the production of excess insulin and amylin is the best way to prevent type 2 diabetes.

It is important to realize that glucose cannot simply diffuse from the blood into the body's cells; it must be shuttled into cells by protein carriers or transporters. There are at least eight different types of glucose transporters found in different tissues in the body. In muscle and fat there are two main types, Glut 1 and Glut 4, that are made in the cell. Glut 1 is normally found in the cell membrane in small numbers and transports a minimal amount of glucose into the muscle cell under basal (without insulin stimulation) conditions. Glut 4 is the insulin-responsive transporter and is normally stored inside the cell. When insulin attaches to the insulin receptor, it signals the cell to move Glut-4 out into the cell membrane where it transports glucose into the cell.

In order to understand what causes the insulin resistance and hyperinsulinemia leading to the pre-diabetic stage, we must first understand how insulin normally works. Figure 4.3 shows how insulin works in skeletal muscle, the most important target tissue for insulin action. When insulin is released from the pancreas into the blood stream, it makes its way to the muscles, where it finds the insulin receptors on the muscle membrane. The insulin receptor consists of four units, two alpha outside the cell where the insulin attaches (binds) and two beta inside the cell. When insulin binds to the alpha subunit, it activates the beta subunit which in turn activates several other factors in the cell (IRS 1/2 and PI3 Kinase) to move the Glut 4 transporters out to the cell membrane to transport glucose into the cell. When insulin resistance develops, there is less activation of the system for any given amount of insulin presented to the receptors, and the body responds by releasing more insulin in an attempt to keep the blood glucose level in the normal range. Most people who are overweight/obese are insulin resistant and have high levels of insulin, which have implications for many health problems that will be discussed in the section on the metabolic syndrome and other diseases. Now that we know how insulin normally works, what causes insulin resistance?

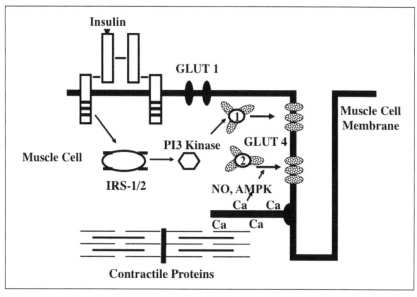

Figure 4.3 Glucose transport regulation in skeletal muscle.

In the 1980s we reported that switching rodents from their normal low-fat, starch diet to a diet high in fat and refined sugar (HFS), similar to the typical U.S. diet, led to insulin resistance and hyperinsulinemia in just 8 weeks.[133] When we looked at the two diet components, fat or sugar, both produced some insulin resistance resulting in hyperinsulinemia, but the combination of both fat and sugar in the diet resulted in the worst effect. Muscles were then isolated to study glucose transport. Basal transport was unaffected by the HFS diet, but insulin-stimulated glucose transport was significantly reduced, indicating insulin resistance. Insulin receptors were then isolated to study activation with insulin. At all levels of insulin, activation of the receptors was

---

[133] American Journal of Physiology, 1987; 252: E420.

reduced in the HFS group. The good news was that switching the animals from the HFS diet back to the low-fat, starch diet for just 4 weeks reversed all of the defects. How exactly the HFS diet causes the decrease in insulin receptor activation is not known but may be the result of increased free radicals and inflammatory cytokines. Recent research by Dr. Olefsky and colleagues at U.C. San Diego has shown that when mice are placed on a high-fat diet, inflammatory cytokines increase in the blood and the mice become insulin resistant.[134] Inflammation will be discussed in detail in Chapter 6.

In addition to the insulin pathway for increasing glucose uptake by muscle cells, there is a second pathway known as the exercise pathway and is shown in Figure 4.3. In order for muscle to contract while we're exercising, our muscle cells release calcium. The calcium also activates our old friend nitric oxide, which induces our cells to move Glut 4 transporters out to the muscle membrane to take up glucose, much as insulin does. Thus, exercise has an insulin-like effect that uses a separate pathway. We initially demonstrated that in rodents a single 45 min bout of treadmill running increased glucose transport into muscle to the same level as did a maximum dose of insulin.[135] Interestingly, although glucose uptake increases with exercise, insulin release from the pancreas is reduced. This effect of exercise to increase glucose uptake by muscle lasts for several hours until glycogen stores are replenished. There is a second phase of increased insulin sensitivity in response to exercise that lasts about 24 hours after the bout of exercise. These results demonstrate the need for daily exercise to optimize blood glucose levels and control insulin resistance. It should be mentioned that although exercise has an insulin-like effect, exercise by itself cannot replace insulin injections in type 1 diabetic patients, but

---

[134] Annual Review of Physiology, 2010; 72: 219.
[135] American Journal of Physiology, 1989; 256: E227.

can reduce the amount of insulin needed to achieve a normal blood glucose level.

Since there are an estimated 57 million individuals in the U.S. with pre-diabetes (and insulin resistance) and only 24 million who are full-blown diabetic, this must mean that not all pre-diabetics will advance to diabetes. This is probably where genetics come into play and is supported by the studies on identical twins. Unfortunately, identifying genetic defects has not been very successful, which suggests that there may be many different genetic defects involved. Regardless of the specific genetic defects that might be involved in type 2 diabetes, the studies on the Pima Indians previously discussed clearly demonstrate that lifestyle plays a more important role in determining whether or not an individual becomes diabetic. This suggests that we need to change the lifestyles of young people in this country to avoid future development of type 2 diabetes. And the sooner we start, the better. Rates of type 2 diabetes are skyrocketing among youth in the U.S. Recent data from the American Diabetes Association show a 21 percent rise in type 2 diabetes rates among U.S. children in just eight years – from 2001 to 2009.[136]

---

[136] Dabelea D et al. Abstract 228-OR. "Is prevalence of type 2 diabetes increasing in youth? The SEARCH for diabetes in Youth Study." American Diabetes Association 72nd Scientific Sessions. Philadelphia: June 8-12, 2012.

Can Type 2 Diabetes be Prevented?

The answer to this question appears to be yes, in most cases. The studies conducted on the Pima Indians discussed earlier showed that the Pimas living in Mexico who were very active physically and consumed a diet of natural foods low in fat and high in fiber had a very low incidence ($\approx$ 10 percent) of type 2 diabetes compared to the Pimas living on the Arizona Reservation ($\approx$ 50 percent) who were inactive and consumed excess calories of the typical U.S. foods along with excess alcohol. In the book *Healthy at 100* by John Robbins, the populations studied were physically active, consumed a natural food diet low in fat and high in fiber, and had almost no diabetes.[137]   In the U.S. Diabetes Prevention Project, 3,234 pre-diabetic individuals were randomized to a control group (taking a placebo), a group taking the drug metformin that increases insulin sensitivity and reduces glucose release from the liver, or thirdly, a group practicing lifestyle change that included low-fat foods and 150 minutes of weekly exercise (brisk walking) with a goal of weight loss. At 2.8 years of average follow-up, the incidence of diabetes compared to placebo was reduced by 31 percent in the metformin group and by 58 percent in the lifestyle group.[138] A similar study conducted in Finland on 522 pre-diabetic individuals also showed the importance of eating more fruits and vegetables combined with 30 minutes of daily exercise. After 3.2 years of follow-up, the intervention group had 27 diabetics (3.3 percent) while the control group had 59 diabetic (7.1 percent) patients.[139] Once again, lifestyle change including diet and exercise was important for preventing diabetes in high-risk

---

[137] Robbins, John. Healthy at 100: The Scientifically Proven Secrets of the World's Healthiest and Longest-Lived Peoples. New York: Ballantine Books, 2007.
[138] New England Journal of Medicine, 2002; 346: 393.
[139] New England Journal of Medicine, 2001; 344: 1343.

individuals. Similar studies conducted in China and Japan showed the same benefits from a healthy diet and exercise.

In view of the discussion of factors that are involved in insulin resistance and the regulation of insulin and its actions, it would not be surprising that the Pritikin Eating Plan, high in complex carbohydrates, antioxidants and fiber, combined with daily exercise, would be more efficacious than drugs in preventing type 2 diabetes, even in high-risk individuals. In several studies we have reported that the Pritikin Program reduces fasting insulin by 30-40 percent,[140] and it was associated with a reduction in calculated insulin resistance. In a recent study we have also found a significant reduction in serum amylin,[141] indicating less chance for amyloid deposits to form and destroy the beta cells leading to type 2 diabetes. Inflammatory cytokines are also significantly reduced by the Pritikin Program and will be discussed in Chapter 6.

How Effective is Lifestyle Change for Treating Type 2 Diabetes?

In the early 1970s Nathan Pritikin met with James Anderson, M.D., at the Kentucky Veterans Administration Hospital to discuss his concept of treating diabetic patients with a high-complex-carbohydrate, high-fiber, low-fat diet, a concept that was revolutionary at the time as most doctors were telling their diabetic patients to avoid carbohydrates. Dr. Anderson agreed to test Mr. Pritikin's diet in the metabolic ward in the hospital using isocaloric diets to rule out any effect of weight loss. Mr. Pritikin didn't like the idea of isocaloric diets as he knew that adopting his diet would normally result in consuming fewer calories due to the low-calorie density and high-fiber

---

[140] Diabetes Research, 2006; 73: 249. Circulation, 2002; 106: 2530. Nutrition and Cancer, 2000: 38: 158.
[141] American Journal of Physiology: Endocrinology & Metabolism, 2012; 303: E542.

content of the food; however, he agreed to Dr. Anderson's plan. In 1976 Dr. Anderson published his first of many papers in the *American Journal of Clinical Nutrition.* The study involved 13 diabetic men, 8 on insulin and 5 on oral agents. After 2 weeks, glucose values fell and all 5 men on oral agents had their medication discontinued. In four men, insulin was discontinued but in 3 men on high doses of insulin (40-55 units), there was little effect of the diet.[142] In 1978 Dr. Anderson published a second paper that involved 10 patients initially treated with the Pritikin diet in the hospital and then followed for an average of 15 months while they continued the diet at home. During the two weeks in the hospital, glucose fell and insulin therapy was discontinued in 5 patients and oral agents discontinued in 3. At follow-up, despite the fact that carbohydrate intake had been reduced from 70 percent of calories in the hospital down to 55-60 percent of calories (still mostly complex), 7 patients remained off medication with no significant rise in glucose.[143]

Dr. Anderson went on to publish several additional papers using the Pritikin diet. In addition to emphasizing the value of the diet for controlling type 2 diabetes, he also pointed out that the diet was effective for lowering cholesterol, triglycerides and blood pressure, all cardiovascular risk factors leading to the number one killer of diabetic patients. In the later 1980s Dr. Anderson served on the American Diabetes Association Nutrition Committee and was instrumental in getting the organization to recommend the high-carbohydrate, high-fiber diet that, unfortunately, was discontinued after a few years when Dr. Anderson left the committee. Over all the years and in his many publications, Dr. Anderson never once mentioned Mr. Pritikin or the Pritikin diet. Later Dr. Anderson admitted that he was told by

---

[142] American Journal of Clinical Nutrition, 1976; 29 (8): 895.
[143] Diabetes Care, 1978; 1: 77.

the Veterans Administration not to include the name Pritikin in his publications.

The experiments conducted by Dr. Anderson in the metabolic ward clearly demonstrated that the Pritikin diet could be important for treating type 2 diabetic patients, especially those on oral agents or low-dose insulin. The experiments involved small numbers and unfortunately did not include exercise, an important component of the Pritikin Program, and an important factor in regulating insulin sensitivity, as discussed earlier. To get more insight into the effectiveness of the Pritikin Program for treating type 2 diabetic patients, I screened the medical charts of 4,587 participants at the Pritikin Longevity Center's 3-week program and found 652 individuals identified as diabetic based on medication or fasting glucose ≥140 mg/dL upon entry. The response to the program is shown in Figure 4.4. The best response was observed in the group on no medication, mostly newly- diagnosed patients, where the glucose was reduced from an average of 164 mg/dL down to 124 mg/dL. Only 5 patients did not respond well and were subsequently placed on oral hypoglycemic agents. The majority (71 percent) of patients initially on oral agents had the drugs discontinued. Of the 212 patients entering the program on insulin, only 39 percent were taken off of insulin, and this was when the glucose level used to define diabetes was 140 mg/dL. Today, the percent having their insulin discontinued would be even lower. This paper was published in *Diabetes Care,* one of the official journals from the American Diabetes Association with the title "Diet and Exercise in the Treatment of NIDDM – The need for early emphasis." The title was obvious from the results. What was not obvious at that time was the underlying mechanism(s). Insulin resistance in muscle and liver had been well documented in type 2 diabetic

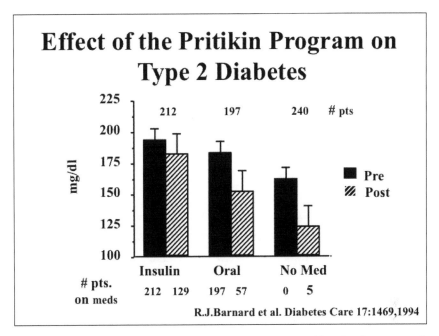

Effect of the Pritikin Program on Type 2 Diabetes

225
212   197   240   # pts
200
175
mg/dl
150   ■ Pre
125   ▨ Post
100

Insulin   Oral   No Med

pts.   212 129   197 57   0   5
on meds

R.J.Barnard et al. Diabetes Care 17:1469,1994

Figure 4.4 Effects of the Pritikin Program on blood glucose and medication in type 2 diabetic patients.[144] When these studies were done, diabetes was defined as a glucose ≥140 mg/dL.

patients, but the reason for the drop in insulin and the fact that patients taking insulin were less likely to respond favorably to the intervention was unknown. As discussed earlier, we now know that the drop in insulin is a result of a reduction in the number of beta, insulin-producing cells in the pancreas. Once the beta cells are destroyed they apparently cannot be regenerated.

In order to assess long-term adherence to the Pritikin Program and to see if any of the patients on insulin were able to discontinue insulin at a later date, indicating possible regeneration of pancreatic beta cells, we contacted a group of 69 patients from our original group 2-3 years after completing the 3-week program at the center. Lipid levels for cholesterol and triglycerides had increased some, but were still significantly below the levels observed at entry into the residential program,

---

[144] Diabetes Care, 1994, 17: 1469.

indicating fairly good adherence to the diet and exercise program.[145] Of the 31 patients initially on oral hypoglycemic agents, there were only 6 on the oral agents at the end of the residential program and at follow-up 7 additional patients were on the oral agents. Of the 18 patients initially on insulin, 12 had the insulin discontinued at the program's end, and at follow-up 4 more were on insulin. Since none of the patients on insulin at the end of the residential program were able to discontinue insulin at follow-up, the results indicate that once beta cells are destroyed, they do not regenerate. We know this is true for type 1 diabetic patients, and it is why scientists are trying to perfect stem cell therapy to re-grow pancreatic beta cells. The fact that beta cells are not regenerated once destroyed makes the title of our paper "Diet and Exercise in the Treatment of NIDDM – The need for early emphasis" even more significant.

The Metabolic Syndrome

Since Dr. Reaven gave the Banting Lecture at the 1988 American Diabetes Association national meeting and introduced the concept of what he called "Syndrome X," now known as the metabolic syndrome (MetS), there has been an exceptional amount of interest in the syndrome with over 31,000 publications and the appearance of a new journal, *The Journal of the CardioMetabolic Syndrome*. The risk factors included in the syndrome described by Dr. Reaven were insulin resistance (hyperinsulinemia or impaired glucose tolerance), hypertension, hypertriglyceridemia, and low, high-density lipoprotein cholesterol (HDL-C), with emphasis on the risk of the syndrome associated with coronary heart disease. Many more factors have been added to the syndrome, and the risk for many different health problems has been suggested, as described in Chapter 1. It has been estimated that 25 percent to 35 percent of all adults in

---

[145] Diabetes Care, 1983; 6: 268

the U.S. have the syndrome and as high as 40 percent of all adults over the age of 60 years have it.[146] Recent studies of obese adolescents in the U.S. suggest that 25 percent may have the syndrome.[147] These statistics make the MetS a serious health issue that is now recognized around the world.

Dr. Reaven, in his Banting Lecture, suggested that insulin resistance and the resultant hyperinsulinemia might be the underlying cause of the syndrome. However, in Chapter 1, I suggested that lifestyle, i.e., diet and lack of exercise, are the true underlying factors responsible for the syndrome. In order to test this hypothesis, a study was conducted on laboratory rats. When rats were raised on a high-fat, refined-sugar diet, similar to the typical U.S. diet, and without any daily exercise, insulin resistance and hyperinsulinemia developed within two weeks.[148] After a few more weeks, the animals showed elevated blood triglyceride levels and after a few more weeks showed enlargement of fat cells indicating fat storage, especially in the abdominal cavity. As time progressed, the animals became hypertensive and displayed increased tendency for blood to clot. None of these problems were observed in the animals raised on a low-fat, complex-carbohydrate diet for up to two years, comparable to a 60-year-old human. This study indicates that diet can induce the MetS, so the obvious question is: Can humans with the syndrome eliminate it with appropriate lifestyle change? To answer this question, a study was conducted on two groups of insulin resistant subjects: one with type 2 diabetes and one with insulin resistance and hyperinsulinemia, but with glucose below the diabetic range (pre-diabetic). These were individuals with the metabolic syndrome attending the Pritikin Longevity Center for 3 weeks. Measurements were taken at the start and end of the

---

[146] JAMA, 2002; 287: 356.
[147] Metabolic Syndrome and Related Disorders, 2013; 11:71.
[148] Journal of Applied Physiology, 1998; 84: 1311.

residential program. Aspects of the syndrome including hyperinsulinemia, hypertension, and hypertriglyceridemia were all reduced.[149] There was a small drop in body weight; however the subjects remained obese, which indicates that obesity is *not* the cause of the syndrome; however, it may exacerbate it. This was one of the first studies to demonstrate that aspects of the MetS could be controlled or eliminated by lifestyle change. It is clear from these studies that the typical U.S. sedentary lifestyle combined with a high-fat, refined carbohydrate, refined-sugar diet induces the syndrome. Furthermore, it is also clear that most aspects of the syndrome can be controlled in a few weeks by undertaking a daily exercise program and consuming a very-low-fat, high-complex-carbohydrate diet built around whole grains, fruits and vegetables, i.e., the Pritikin Eating Plan. In a recent publication, we reported that 7 overweight/obese children attending the Pritikin Family Program entered with the MetS. After just two weeks of the Pritikin Program, all 7 had reduced their insulin, triglycerides and blood pressure, and were no longer classified as having the MetS.[150] In a study of 67 adults with MetS who attended the Pritikin Longevity Center, 37 percent of the subjects were no longer classified as having the syndrome after just two weeks at the Center.[151] While Dr. Reaven was probably correct when he suggested that insulin resistance and hyperinsulinemia were underlying factors for the other aspects of the syndrome, including hypertension and hypertriglyceridemia, he failed to take the discussion one step further to point out that the typical U.S. lifestyle was the true underlying cause of the MetS.

---

[149] Journal of Applied Physiology, 2006; 100: 1657.
[150] Metabolism Clinical and Experimental, 2006; 55: 871.
[151] Journal of the CardioMetabolic Syndrome, 2006; 1: 308.

Chapter 5

Cancer – The # 2 Killer in the U.S.

While mortality from cardiovascular disease has been reduced substantially during the past 40 years, mortality from cancer has increased. However, in very recent times mortality from cancer has also decreased, resulting in an increase in life expectancy. Radiation, chemotherapy, and other drugs or surgical treatments are usually effective for a period of time, but most patients eventually die with cancer. Unfortunately, little progress has been made in the prevention field. The reason this is unfortunate is the fact that the vast majority of cancers are lifestyle related.[152] The one exception in the prevention field is breast cancer, where both the incidence and mortality have decreased in the past few years, thought to be due in large part to the discontinued use of hormone treatment in postmenopausal women. In addition to the lifestyle factors of poor diet, smoking and lack of exercise, all of which are also related to cardiovascular disease, exposure to chemical carcinogens is another important aspect of cancer development that has received little attention (except for cigarette smoke).

Cancer is characterized by uncontrolled cell growth that results in the formation of a tumor. Two types of tumors may form in the body, benign or malignant (cancerous). A benign tumor is simply a mass of abnormal cells growing in a tissue. The cells may be encapsulated in a connective tissue cover and simply occupy space. When they grow to the size where they are painful or unsightly, they may be removed. Some benign tumors

---

[152] World Cancer Research Fund/American Institute for Cancer Research. Food, Nutrition, Physical Activity and the Prevention of Cancer: a Global Perspective. Washington, DC: AICR, 2007.

may undergo further mutations and become malignant tumors; intestinal polyps are an example. Malignant or cancerous tumors do more than occupy space. They destroy the normal tissue where they reside, and, because they are not encapsulated, pieces break off and enter the blood stream or lymph system and move to other parts of the body where they begin to grow. This process is known as metastasis and usually results in cancer death.

How Does Cancer Develop?

Figure 5.1 shows a theory on cancer development. It starts with damage to the genetic material, the DNA, contained in the nucleus of the cells. A carcinogen or other factors including virus, radiation, or inflammation damage the DNA, creating a pre-neoplastic, or abnormal, cell. In some cases the damaged DNA may simply be due to random chance as cells undergo division and replication stimulated by genes normally present in the body (oncogenes) that become over active. Some recent studies indicate that cancer is not actually caused by damage to the DNA code itself but by damage inflicted on the proteins that

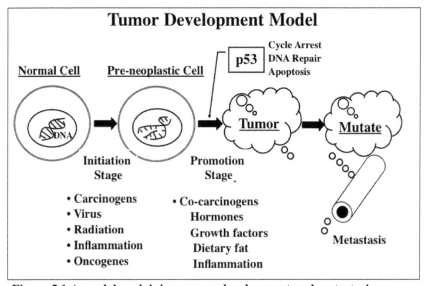

Figure 5.1 A model explaining cancer development and metastasis.

are attached to the DNA strands and turn on or turn off the DNA replication process. More and more studies emphasize the role of inflammation in many common cancers. Studies of people who take aspirin on a regular basis to reduce inflammation in arthritic joints and/or blood clotting in CAD patients show reduced risk for most of the major cancers including lung, breast, prostate, and colo/rectal.[153] As we are all exposed on a daily basis to many factors that can damage DNA, most of us have a number of pre-neoplastic cells in our body at any one time. The body has a defense mechanism in a gene known as p53. This gene surveys the DNA genome, and if it detects a defect or mutation, it should immediately activate other genes to halt cell division, repair the defect, or program the cell to die (apoptosis). However, because cancer is so common in our society, it is obvious that the p53 gene is not always effective. As we will learn later, the p53 gene is suppressed by factors related to lifestyle. The pre-neoplastic cell may be stimulated by a co-carcinogen and start to divide. This is known as the promotion stage and results in the formation of a tumor. Some co-carcinogens have been identified, including hormones such as estrogen, testosterone, and insulin, growth factors such as insulin-like growth factor (IGF-1), inflammation, and dietary fat.

Of the most common solid-tumor (as opposed to blood cancers) cancers, lung, breast, prostate and colo/rectal, the underlying cause is best understood for lung cancer. It is well documented that smoking or being exposed to second-hand smoke provides the carcinogens to cause cancer. According to the National Cancer Institute, smoking causes 87 percent of all lung cancer. At least 60 chemical carcinogens are associated with tobacco. Exposure to second-hand smoke increases the risk for lung cancer by 30 percent. Tobacco use is also responsible for cancers other than lung, including cancer of the oral cavity,

---

[153] The Lancet, 2012; 379: 1602.

pharynx, larynx, esophagus, and bladder. Another chemical carcinogen associated with lung cancer is asbestos and is especially dangerous if combined with cigarette smoke. Additionally, there are more than 80,000 man-made chemicals approved for use in the U.S. and in most cases their impact on health, including cancer, is unknown. Recent studies report that the use of common pesticides increases the risk for certain cancers.[154] Studies on migrant farm workers show increased risk for several different cancers.[155] Recent data reported for U.S. soldiers exposed to the pesticide agent orange in Viet Nam show increased incidence of more aggressive prostate cancer at younger ages.[156] Studies on wives of Midwest farmers show increased incidence of breast cancer.[157]

Viruses have been linked to certain forms of cancer. For example, hepatitis B & C have been linked to liver cancer. *Helicobacter pylori,* an underlying cause of stomach ulcers, has also been linked to stomach cancer, papilloma viruses have been linked to cancers of the cervix, anus, penis, and vagina. Epstein-Barr virus has also been shown to increase the risk for several different cancers. Viruses are thought to cause cancer by altering cellular DNA and/or by inducing inflammation. Chronic inflammatory bowel diseases such as ulcerative colitis increase the risk for colo/rectal cancer. Inflammation is also thought to play a role in lung cancer and in the early stages of breast and prostate cancer development even before the tissue becomes truly cancerous. Chronic inflammation, especially as related to lifestyle, will be discussed in detail in Chapter 6.

---

[154] Gold, L.S, et al. Pesticide Residues in Food and Cancer Risk: A Critical Analysis. In: Handbook of Pesticide Toxicology. San Diego, California: Academic Press, 2001.
[155] Journal of Agromedicine, 2009; 14: 185.
[156] Cancer, 2013; 119: 2399.
[157] American Journal of Epidemiology, 2005; 161 (2): 121.

Radiation is also known to damage DNA and lead to cancer. Of special concern is excessive exposure to the ultraviolet rays from the sun or from tanning beds. Although exposure to the sun (15-20 minutes daily) is important for vitamin D formation, longer exposures increase the risk for the deadly skin cancer melanoma. According to the World Health Organization, the scientific evidence linking indoor tanning to the deadly skin cancer melanoma is "sufficient and compelling."[158]

The initiation of cancer that starts with a normal cell and progresses through the pre-neoplastic stage may involve up to fifteen different changes or mutations in the cell before it becomes truly neoplastic. During this period of time, the p53 gene should be activated to stop the process by blocking cell division, repairing the damaged DNA, or inducing the cell to go into apoptosis (cell death). However several factors, mostly lifestyle related, can block the action of the p53 gene. One of these is the growth factor insulin-like growth factor-1 (IGF-I). Studies conducted by Dr. Derek LeRoith and his colleagues at the National Institutes of Health showed that cells grown in culture and damaged by certain chemicals known as UV-mimetics would activate the p53 gene to induce apoptosis. However, if they added IGF-I to the cell cultures, p53 in the cell was decreased and the cells survived with the damaged DNA.[159] Other studies have shown that IGF-I added to cancer cells stimulates growth and blocks apoptosis. Not surprisingly, IGF-I has been reported in epidemiological studies to be a risk factor for several cancers, including breast, prostate, colon, and lung.

Dietary fat is another factor known to promote cancer formation and progression. Studies conducted as far back as the 1940s demonstrated a link between dietary fat and cancer

---

[158] World Health Organization's International Agency for Research on Cancer, special report on radiation, The Lancet Oncology, 2009; 10: 751.
[159] The Journal of Biological Chemistry, 2002; 277: 15600.

development. When rodents were given a chemical known to induce cancer and then placed on different fat diets, the number of animals that developed tumors over the period of observation was twice as high on the high-fat diets. It didn't matter that the fat content of the diet was increased by adding animal fat (saturated fat), vegetable oil (primarily polyunsaturated fat), or mono-unsaturated oil, tumor development was increased.[160] As discussed in Chapter 1, epidemiological studies have reported a relationship between total dietary fat intake and cancer incidence for most of the common cancers.

Exactly how the fat content of the diet induces the development of tumors is not known, but there are several possibilities. First, as discussed in Chapter 4, high-fat diets induce insulin resistance, resulting in serum hyperinsulinemia. Insulin is a known anabolic hormone that stimulates cell growth and has been shown to increase tumor cell growth in culture. In addition to directly stimulating tumor cell growth, insulin is also known to stimulate the liver to produce IGF-I. As described above, elevated IGF-I stimulates growth as well as blocks apoptosis in tumor cells by blocking the p53 gene. Dietary fat, especially saturated fat, stimulates inflammatory cytokine production that also stimulates growth and blocks apoptosis of tumor cells. Insulin also blocks liver production of sex hormone-binding globulin (SHBG), a protein that binds both male and female sex hormones and limits their availability to stimulate estrogen and/or testosterone receptors. Reduced levels of SHBG result in increased hormone action that is crucial for the development of breast and prostate cancers.

Once tumors develop and start to grow, a process that might take many years depending on the type of cancer, cells may break from the tumor and enter the blood stream or lymphatic system to spread to other parts of the body

---

[160] Cancer Research, 1943; 3: 749.

(metastasis). Also during this period of time, the tumor might acquire additional changes or mutations. This may be in response to certain treatments or may simply be the nature of the tumor as not all tumors in the same tissue have the same genetic defects. For example, nearly all early-stage cancers have an intact p53 gene, but it is suppressed by factors like IGF-I, as described above. Some tumors, as they acquire further mutations, may develop defects in the p53 gene itself that render it ineffective and usually results in an aggressive tumor.

Prostate Cancer

The prostate gland, part of the urogenital system in males, is about the size of a walnut and is located just below the bladder, wrapping around the urethra (the tube running from the bladder to the penis). The function of the prostate gland is to produce, store and secrete a slightly alkaline fluid during ejaculation. Prostate cancer (PCa) is by far the most common solid-tumor cancer in Western men. According to a study of 44,788 pairs of twins from Denmark, Finland, and Sweden, almost 60 percent of the PCa was attributable to environmental/lifestyle factors.[161] Of the remaining 40 percent that was attributable to inheritance, it has to be kept in mind that lifestyle may still be an important factor, as was previously discussed with type 2 diabetes. Put simply, a genetic susceptibility to a cancer can be "activated" by our lifestyle choices. Prostate cancer has been proposed to start as a condition where inflammation causes atrophy of the prostate epithelial cells (cells that line the ducts in the prostate gland) and begins to damage the genetic material. Further genetic damage results in the development of prostatic intraepithelial neoplasia (uncontrolled epithelial cell growth), eventually leading to prostate cancer. In the early stages, all PCa is androgen-dependent, which means that testosterone must be present for the

---

[161] New England Journal of Medicine, 2000; 343: 78.

cancer to develop. Men who are castrated early in life or who are born with genetic defects that prohibit the production or action of testosterone never get PCa. Some men who develop PCa are treated by hormone therapy (androgen deprivation) to shrink the tumors. This treatment initially involved surgical castration, but more recently drugs are used to reduce testosterone production or to block its action at the receptor. This treatment is commonly used when the cancer has spread from the prostate to other parts of the body. After the tumor shrinks and the disease is regressed for a period of time, the tumors might start to grow again and generally become androgen-independent tumors that are very aggressive. On the other hand, if the disease is detected early and treated, long-term survival is usually quite good. Obviously, an important question is: What is the best way to detect PCa in its early stages?

Early-stage PCa is usually not accompanied by any symptoms, so men have to rely on regular medical exams for detection, including a digital rectal exam (DRE) and blood test for prostate-specific antigen (PSA). The DRE is the old finger in the rectum and should be part of a regular physical exam for men. PSA is a protein produced by the prostate gland and released into the blood. The values are normally very low, less than 4 ng/mL. However, with PCa development they generally rise. PSA was discovered in the mid 1980s and greatly increased the number of men diagnosed with PCa, but there are limitations to both the DRE and the PSA tests as neither is close to 100 percent accurate. These tests can have abnormal results even when PCa is not present (false positive) or can have normal results when PCa is present (false negative). False results can lead to some men undergoing unneeded biopsies with risk of pain, infection and/or bleeding, or may give men a false sense of security when they actually have PCa. It is obvious that better screening tests are needed to more accurately detect PCa.

There is no question that the PSA test can spot many early prostate cancers. However, there is great concern that once detected, many men undergo invasive treatment for their PCa that may not be needed, especially in much older men. Due to the fact that most PCa progresses slowly, it has recently been recommended that men at age 75 who have a normal PSA test should no longer have the test on an annual basis as is presently recommended.[162] Another challenge to the medical community is to develop tests capable of detecting tumor biopsies showing that the tumors are likely to grow more rapidly and be more aggressive. The alternative is to place men with PCa on "watchful waiting" and measure their PSA every 6 months and watch the doubling time as an indicator of aggressiveness of the disease.

PCa and the Pritikin Program

Over the past ten-plus years an extensive amount of research relative to PCa has been conducted on men attending the Pritikin Longevity Center. Data published in over 17 scientific papers and 5 review articles clearly support the hypothesis that the Pritikin Program should be effective for preventing PCa as well as being important for the treatment of early PCa. While doing research on the impact of diet on insulin resistance as described in Chapter 4, several papers appeared in the scientific literature indicating that high levels of insulin depress liver production of sex hormone-binding globulin (SHBG), resulting in elevated levels of free estradiol and testosterone. As previously reported, a study was conducted to measure both serum insulin and SHBG in men attending the Pritikin Longevity Center program. As expected, insulin was reduced by 43 percent and SHBG was increased by 38 percent.[163] In a follow-up study, we measured testosterone in a group of men. Total testosterone was

[162] Annals of Internal Medicine, 2012; 157: 120.
[163] Nutrition and Cancer, 1998; 31: 127.

unchanged but free testosterone (testosterone not bound to a protein to render it inactive) was reduced by 19 percent in response to the program and rise in SHBG.[164] These first studies suggested that the Pritikin Program might be important for prevention and/or treatment of PCa and encouraged us to do additional studies.

It is well known that tumors in the body must develop a blood supply in order to survive. This indicates that circulating blood (serum) factors might have an important influence on growth and survival of the tumors. To test the hypothesis that the Pritikin Program could alter serum factors that may influence the growth and survival of tumor cells, we developed a unique bioassay. Prostate cancer cells were grown in culture and stimulated with serum obtained from men attending the Pritikin Program. In the first study, serum samples were obtained from 13 men attending the two-week program, meaning the time between the in- and out-going serum samples was only eleven days. When the serum samples were used to stimulate PCa cells for two days, the growth rate was reduced by 35 percent in the post- compared to the pre-serum samples.[165] These studies were done using androgen-dependent PCa cells that would be indicative of early stage PCa. The results were confirmed with a second androgen-dependent PCa cell line.[166] However, when studies were done using androgen-independent PCa cells, indicative of end-stage PCa, there was very little reduction in growth with the Pritikin Program serum. Bottom Line: Early action appears vital. If a man waits till late-stage prostate cancer to adopt a healthy lifestyle, it may, unfortunately, be too late.

In order to assess the long-term effects of following the Pritikin Program, serum samples were obtained from some of the

---

[164] Nutrition and Cancer, 2002; 42: 112.
[165] Journal of Urology, 2001; 166: 1185.
[166] Clinical Cancer Research, 2003; 9: 2734.

Longevity Center staff members who had been following the program for an average of 14 years. The results showed that compared to men entering the Pritikin Program, the serum from the staff members had a 45 percent reduction in the growth rate of androgen-dependent PCa cells.[167] In an attempt to identify factors that changed in the serum as a result of the Pritikin Program that might reduce the growth of the tumor cells, we selected insulin, testosterone and estradiol, factors previously shown to be reduced by the Pritikin Program. We first demonstrated that each of these serum factors independently would stimulate the growth of PCa cells. However, when we added all three back to the post-program serum, at the concentrations shown to be reduced by the program, we could account for less than half of the reduction in growth of the PCa cells observed with the Pritikin Program serum.[168] These results suggested that other factors were also changing in the serum that could affect the growth of the tumor cells.

Several epidemiological studies had reported that the growth factor IGF-I was a risk factor for PCa. Also, at about the same time, Dr. LeRoith and his colleagues at the National Institutes of Health published data showing that IGF-I would block the actions of the p53 gene in cells with damaged DNA. In addition, other papers reported that IGF-I added to cultured cancer cells stimulated growth and blocked apoptosis (cell death). Thus, we decided to investigate the effects of the Pritikin Program on serum IGF-I and one of its binding proteins IGFBP-1. If we have higher levels of IGFBP-1, we have less active IGF-I. The results showed that after two weeks at the Pritikin Longevity Center, not only was serum IGF-I reduced by 20 percent but IGFBP-1 was increased by 53 percent.[169] The serum

---

[167] Journal of Urology, 2001; 166: 1185.
[168] Nutrition and Cancer, 2002; 42: 112
[169] Cancer Causes & Control, 2002; 13: 929.

from the Longevity Center staff men (long-term compliers) had IGF-I levels that were 55 percent lower than the levels for the men entering the Pritikin Program, and IGFBP-1 levels were 150 percent higher. When all of the data were combined (pre, post, long term), serum IGF-I was positively correlated with PCa cell growth while IGFBP-1 was negatively correlated, meaning, the higher the levels of IGF-1 in the blood, the greater the cancer growth; and the lower the levels of IGFBP-1, the more cancer cell growth.

More important than the reduction in PCa cell growth found with the Pritikin Program serum was the discovery that cell death (apoptosis) was increased. Serum samples from the men entering the Pritikin Program showed almost no apoptosis, and that explains, in part, why PCa is so common in U.S. men. Following 11 days of the Pritikin Program, apoptosis was dramatically increased in the cell culture studies and was even greater in the studies with serum from the Pritikin staff with long-term compliance to the program.[170] Studies conducted with an androgen-independent PCa cell line showed no significant increase in apoptosis following the Pritikin Program. These results indicate that the Pritikin Program should be effective for prevention and treatment of early PCa but would be of much lesser value for treating advanced, androgen-independent PCa.

To test the efficacy of lifestyle change, including a 10-percent fat-calorie diet and daily exercise for treating early-stage PCa, we teamed with Dr. Dean Ornish to study a group of men diagnosed with early PCa who were placed on "watchful waiting." This was a randomized study with 44 men in the lifestyle treatment group and 49 in the control group who received standard medical care from their personal physicians. Over the first year, serum prostate specific antigen (PSA), a marker for PCa, increased in the control group from 6.4 to 6.7

---

[170] Cancer Causes & Control, 2002; 13: 929.

ng/mL but decreased in the experimental group from 6.2 to 6.0 ng/mL.[171] While the changes in PSA were not impressive, the clinical outcomes were impressive. At one year, 6 men in the control group had received conventional treatment (on advice from their physician), including prostatectomy, radiation, androgen deprivation, or brachytherapy due to rising PSA or MRI results indicating advancing disease. None of the men in the experimental group had signs of advancing PCa and thus did not require aggressive treatment. Serum samples obtained at the start and after one year from both groups were used in our bioassay to stimulate PCa cells. Growth with the control-group serum was reduced by 9 percent while the experimental group serum showed a 70 percent reduction in PCa cell growth after one year. What was surprising was the fact that there was only a small increase in apoptosis that was observed in both the control and experimental groups. This was at first puzzling until we were informed that the men in the experimental group were given soy protein supplements to take daily. Several reports in the literature indicate that high-quality protein, like soy, increases serum IGF-I. When we measured serum IGF-I levels in the men taking the soy supplements, we found that it had increased from 168 to 199 ng/mL, and that may have accounted for the lack of a significant increase in apoptosis in the bioassay as IGF-I blocks the p53 gene and apoptosis as explained earlier. To further test the hypothesis that high soy protein intake would increase serum IGF-I and block apoptosis in the bioassay, we conducted a clinical trial at UCLA in the Clinical Research Center where for one month all meals were provided to men with PCa who were scheduled for surgery.[172] The low-fat diet (15 percent calories) was achieved by increasing the protein content (up to 30 percent calories) including 35 gm of soy protein daily. Again, the growth rate of

---

[171] Journal of Urology, 2005; 174: 1065.
[172] Journal of Urology, 2010; 183: 345.

the PCa cells in the serum-stimulated bioassay was reduced with the low-fat diet, but there was no increase in apoptosis. This was a surprise so we measured serum IGF-I and found that it had increased from 241 to 299 ng/mL, confirming other studies showing that high protein intake, especially from soy, increases serum IGF-I and blocks apoptosis. Based on the results from these two studies, the Pritikin Program does not recommend soy supplements or high-protein diets in general, especially for men with PCa.

From this discussion it appears that the reduction in serum IGF-I resulting from the Pritikin Program would be of prime importance for reducing growth and inducing apoptosis in prostate tumor cells and would be important for preventing and/or treating early-stage PCa. To test this hypothesis, studies were conducted using the cell cultures of androgen-dependent PCa cells and adding IGF-I back to the post-Pritikin serum samples. The results showed that adding back the IGF-I completely blocked the decrease in tumor cell growth as well as the increase in apoptosis observed following the Pritikin Program.[173] To further confirm the importance of reducing serum IGF-I for reducing tumor cell growth and inducing apoptosis, we measured the p53 content in the tumor cells and found that in the post serum-stimulated cells, the p53 content was doubled. We also measured p21, a gene activated by p53 that blocks the tumor cells from dividing, and found that it was also doubled in the post serum-stimulated cancer cells.[174] In view of the results from the cell culture studies as well as the clinical results from the Ornish prostate cancer treatment study, we wanted to find out: Could lifestyle changes actually alter the biochemistry of the prostate gland? The answer is yes, lifestyle changes, including diet, can directly affect the cancerous prostate gland. Initial studies

---

[173] Endocrinology, 2003; 144: 2319.
[174] European Journal of Cancer Prevention, 2007; 16: 415.

conducted on patients with PCa in which biopsies were obtained before and after lifestyle change clearly show changes in prostate cell membranes as well as alterations in prostate gene expression that would favor reduced risk and/or a more favorable clinical outcome.

As all of the data previously discussed clearly indicate that the Pritikin Program should be important for the prevention and/or early treatment of PCa, we wanted to find out what might be more important: the diet or the daily exercise. We obtained serum samples from men attending the UNLV Adult Fitness Program where they exercised five days a week for one hour with no dietary intervention and compared the results in the bioassay with results obtained with serum from the Pritikin Program staff members and from control men with no diet intervention or

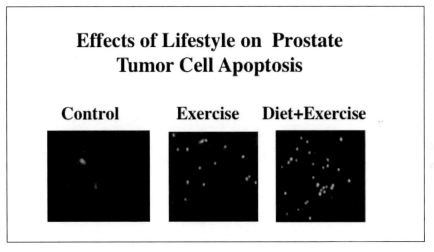

Figure 5.2 Prostate cancer cells programmed to die (apoptosis) following 2 days of incubation in serum from men with different lifestyle attributes. The bright green cells are all the cells in the culture that are signaling apoptosis.

exercise.[175] The reduction in PCa cell growth and increase in apoptosis observed in the Pritikin subjects compared to the

---

[175] Prostate, 2003; 56: 201.

control men were dramatic, as previously discussed. The results with the serum from the UNLV men with only exercise were half as good as the results from the Pritikin men, confirming the importance of daily exercise combined with a healthy diet. Figure 5.2 demonstrates the impact of lifestyle on PCa cell apoptosis. After 2 days of incubation in serum from the control men, there was almost no apoptosis in the PCa cells while the serum from the UNLV men (exercise only) and the Pritikin men (diet and exercise) dramatically increased apoptosis with the Pritikin samples showing superior results.

Benign Prostatic Hyperplasia (BPH) and the Pritikin Program

BPH is a very common condition in older men, affecting up to 80 percent of U.S. men over the age of 80 yrs. BPH often leads to a condition known as LUTS (lower urinary tract symptoms) that includes frequent urination, especially at night, and urgency or other urinary problems that may require medication or even surgery. BPH may or may not be associated with prostate cancer. Many men with BPH never get PCa; however, men with PCa generally also have BPH, suggesting some relationship even though the two conditions generally develop in different areas of the prostate gland. The only two established factors associated with BPH are age and testosterone. Aging itself cannot be a causative factor, and with aging, testosterone levels decline, suggesting that other factors are involved in stimulating growth of the prostate gland in older men.

Recent studies have suggested that elevated serum levels of estradiol, insulin and insulin-like growth factor (IGF-I) may be involved in stimulating growth of the prostate, leading to benign prostatic hyperplasia (BPH), commonly referred to as enlarged prostate. As we have published several papers showing reductions in these factors in men attending the Pritikin Center, we postulated that the serum changes might reduce the growth of prostate tissue that leads to BPH. Thus, a study was conducted with serum obtained from men attending the Pritikin Center.[176] The serum was used to stimulate prostate epithelial cells grown in cultures. The results showed that the Pritikin Program altered serum factors that reduced the growth of the epithelial cells but did not affect apoptosis of the cells. These results suggest that the Pritikin Program might slow the growth of the prostate gland to reduce BPH and the development of lower urinary tract symptoms (LUTS).

Breast Cancer

Breast cancer (BCa), like PCa, is a hormone-dependent cancer. In BCa the hormones responsible are estrogens (mainly estradiol) as opposed to androgens (testosterone) in the case of PCa. Despite the fact that different hormones are responsible, many of the genetic defects identified in the two cancers are similar. There are also other similarities between the two cancers. For example, insulin and IGF-I are risk factors for both cancers. Also, the international variation in the incidence of both cancers are similar, and the variations correlate with dietary fat consumption, that is, the countries with the highest dietary fat intake also tend to have the highest incidences of both breast and prostate cancer.[177] Obesity and a lack of exercise are also risk factors for both cancers. Migration studies for both cancers show that when individuals from low-incidence countries move to high-incidence countries, i.e., the U.S., the incidence of both cancers increase,[178] supporting the contention that lifestyle is a major factor in both cancers. In addition, inflammation is thought to be involved in the early stages of both cancers and is related to consumption of dietary fat, as will be discussed in Chapter 6.

---

[176] Prostate Cancer & Prostatic Diseases, 2008; 11: 362.
[177] International Journal of Cancer, 1975; 15: 617.
[178] International Journal of Cancer, 1975; 15: 617. Journal of the National Cancer Institute, 1993; 85: 1819.

Despite the fact that BCa is typically an estrogen-dependent cancer, most BCa in the developed countries occurs after menopause, when estrogen and related ovarian hormones are no longer produced by the ovaries, and the serum levels of the estrogens drop dramatically. Many speculate that early life exposure of the breast tissue to estrogens may be a significant factor in determining the risk for BCa after menopause. In countries with very low incidences of BCa, where people follow traditional diets low in fat, females do not experience menarche until late in the teens and go into menopause in the late 40s compared to the U.S., where menarche is experienced earlier, around age 10, and menopause later, usually after age 50. Recent data published in *Pediatrics* found that 15 percent of 7 year olds in the U.S. were experiencing puberty.[179] The exact reason for the early onset of menarche is not known, but some have speculated that exposure to estrogen-like chemicals found in many plastic products and some pesticides could be involved. The early onset of menarche and late menopause, in addition to higher levels of estrogens throughout the menstrual cycle, greatly increase the lifetime exposure of the breast tissue to estrogen and is associated with increased risk for BCa in the developed countries.

When women go into menopause and the ovaries stop producing estrogens, the level of estrogens in the serum does not drop to zero, as estrogen continues to be produced in fat cells through the action of an enzyme known as aromatase. This enzyme converts androgens and other steroid hormones from the adrenal gland to estrogen. Studies with isolated fat cells from women have shown that insulin and/or inflammatory cytokines stimulate aromatase activity to increase estrogen production.[180] Thus, it is not surprising that obese, hyperinsulinemic women

---

[179] Pediatrics, 2010; 126; e583.
[180] Journal of Clinical Investigation, 1983; 72: 1150.

who have higher levels of inflammatory cytokines and estrogen are at increased risk for BCa.

In addition to the fat tissue-produced estrogen, many women have taken estrogen hormone therapy after menopause. In the 1990s almost all major health and physician organizations encouraged post-menopausal women to take hormones mainly to prevent coronary heart disease, the number one killer of women. This was initially referred to as hormone replacement therapy (HRT) but was really a misnomer as the hormones given to women were equine estrogen and progestin (synthetic progesterone) that were not truly replacement of natural human hormones. The term HRT was later replaced with hormone therapy (HT). The advice for women to take the HT was given on the basis of some observational studies and the known fact that pre-menopausal women do not show clinical signs of heart disease. Since far more women die from heart attacks than from BCa, physicians were willing to take the risk with HT to save more lives. Finally, the National Institute of Health in 1991 commissioned a large randomized study to evaluate the overall effects of HT on women's health. The study, termed the Women's Health Initiative, was designed to be a 15-year study but was stopped early in 2002 due to increased mortality and morbidity in the HT group.[181] As expected, there was an increase in diagnosed BCa in the HT group compared to placebo, but the increase of 26 percent was greater than expected. What was *not* expected was an increase in coronary events of 30 percent, an increase in strokes of 41 percent and an increase in thromboembolism (clots) of 111 percent in the HT group. There was a 34 percent reduction in the incidence of hip fractures, as expected, as estrogen is important for bone formation. In the year 2000, 46 million prescriptions were written for HT. This number has been dramatically reduced and is thought to be a major factor

---

[181] JAMA, 2002; 288 (3): 321.

in the reductions in BCa diagnosis and mortality recently observed in the U.S. However, a recent German study concluded that HT, as well as a lack of exercise, are still the major factors responsible for most BCa.[182]

Effect of the Pritikin Program on Estrogen and BCa Risk

In 1990 we sent serum samples from thirteen obese, postmenopausal women attending the Pritikin 3-week program to Dr. David Heber, Chief of Clinical Nutrition at the UCLA School of Medicine, to measure estradiol. The results were amazing. In just three weeks Dr. Heber found a 50 percent decrease in serum estradiol in the postmenopausal women.[183] These results were confirmed in a later study in postmenopausal women attending the 2-week Pritikin Program.[184] Not only did women not on HT respond with a decrease in estradiol (37 percent) but also women on HT responded favorably with a 34 percent decrease in estradiol. The decreases observed in this 2-week study were accompanied with a 40 percent increase in sex hormone-binding globulin (SHBG) indicating a decrease in the amount of free estrogen available to stimulate the breast tissue. The observed decreases in serum estradiol with the two- or three-week intervention must be due to changes in estradiol metabolism in the body as the subjects were still overweight or obese after the reductions in estradiol.

The reductions in estradiol could be due to the observed reductions in insulin and inflammatory cytokines known to stimulate aromatase activity and estradiol production in fat cells. Another factor could be enhanced estrogen excretion as a result of the high-fiber content of the Pritikin diet.

In yet another study of postmenopausal women attending the Longevity Center for two weeks, we confirmed the reduction

---

[182] Cancer Epidemiology, 2011; 35 (4): 345.
[183] Nutrition, 1991; 7: 137.
[184] Nutrition and Cancer, 2000; 38: 158. Jim:

in estradiol.[185] In addition, we measured the growth factor IGF-I, as it had been reported to be a risk factor for BCa. IFG-I was reduced by 19 percent while the binding protein (IGFBP-1) was increased by 32 percent. Recall from the discussion on PCa, the higher the IGFBP-1 and lower the IGF-I, the lower the tumor cell growth. Serum samples from twelve of the women were used in our bioassay with three estrogen-receptor positive BCa cell lines. In all three cell lines, serum-stimulated growth was reduced and apoptosis (programmed cell death) was significantly increased with the post-program samples.

Although most clinical BCa occurs in postmenopausal women in the U.S., *the lifetime* exposure to estrogens is thought to be a major factor in determining BCa risk, as discussed earlier. Thus, in collaboration with Dr. Heber at UCLA, we conducted a clinical trial with pre-menopausal women.[186] Twelve women age 25-45 years, not on birth-control pills and with normal menstrual function and normal weight, were recruited from UCLA. The study was conducted through the UCLA General Clinical Research Center, where all major meals were prepared and distributed to the subjects. During the first month, the women were stabilized on a diet with 30 percent of calories from fat and 15-20 g of fiber per day, as recommended by major health organizations for disease prevention. After recording baseline data, the women were placed on a diet with 10 percent of calories from fat and 25-35 g of fiber per day for two months, following the Pritikin guidelines. During the two months on the Pritikin diet, the women lost a small amount of weight while total length of the menstrual cycle and duration of the two phases were unchanged. Compared to the 30 percent fat-calorie baseline diet, the Pritikin diet resulted in a 25 percent decrease in estradiol during the follicular phase and a 22 percent decrease during the

---

185   Nutrition and Cancer, 2006; 55: 28.
186   Cancer, 1995; 76: 2491.

luteal phase. Estrone (another estrogen) was reduced by 19 and 18 percent during the follicular and luteal phases of the cycle, respectfully, following adoption of the Pritikin diet. These results indicate that long-term compliance to the Pritikin lifestyle during the pre-menopausal period would reduce estrogen levels and should reduce the risk for BCa.

Colon Cancer

Colon cancer, also known as colo/rectal cancer (CRCa), includes cancerous growths in the colon (large intestines), rectum (end of the intestines), or appendix. CRCa is the third leading cause of cancer deaths in both men and women in the U.S. CRCa is thought to start with inflammation of the epithelial cells that line the insides of the intestines. This leads to the development of benign tumors known as adenomatous polyps. With further mutations the polyps become cancerous tissue. Chronic inflammatory bowel diseases such as ulcerative colitis increase the risk for colorectal cancer. Inflammation might also be related to dietary factors. CRCa usually provides no overt symptoms, especially in the early stages. Thus, it is important to have regular medical exams such as a colonoscopy that can detect the benign polyps before they become cancerous.

Like prostate and breast cancers, there is a large international variation in mortality from CRCa that correlates with dietary fat.[187] The correlation with dietary fat is not surprising as dietary fat, especially saturated fat, induces inflammation and will be discussed in detail in Chapter 6. Another factor that can induce inflammation is increased bile acids, especially secondary bile acids. As discussed in Chapter 2, bile is formed in the liver from the breakdown of cholesterol, is stored in the gall bladder, and following consumption of a high-fat meal, is released into the intestines to aid in the digestion and

---

[187] International Journal of Cancer, 1975; 15: 617.

absorption of fat particles into the body. Think of bile acids as the detergent in your digestive systems. And just as you need *more* detergent when dealing with greasy fat-encrusted pots and pans, you need more detergent, or bile, when dealing with your body's intake of high-fat meals. The primary bile acids formed in the liver may be converted into secondary bile acids by the anaerobic microbial flora in the intestines. Secondary bile acids have been shown to be carcinogenic as have the anaerobic flora, both of which are increased with a diet high in fat and protein.

Another dietary factor that may play an important role in preventing CRCa is fiber and is found in all plant foods. It is not digested and thus passes through the GI system ending in the feces. Dietary fiber is divided into soluble or insoluble fiber. Both are important for good health, preventing/relieving constipation. Insoluble fibers are found in whole-wheat flour and many vegetables. They increase stool bulk and increase movement of material through the GI tract, reducing transit time. Soluble fibers are found in oats, beans and many fruits and vegetables. They dissolve in water to form a gel-like material. Both types of fiber are abundant in the Pritikin Eating Plan. One of the first individuals to suggest that dietary fiber might play a role in CRCa and other GI problems was Dr. Burkitt, a British-trained physician who moved to South Africa to practice medicine. He immediately noticed a dramatic difference in GI problems between the African villagers and the British residents and suggested that removing fiber by processing carbohydrates was related to increased CRCa in the British population. In 1969 he published the results of a study[188] conducted with a group of British and a group of African villagers where he measured transit time (the time to pass through the GI tract) and stool weight as he noticed the African villagers appeared to have bigger and looser stools. The transit time for the British group

---

[188] Lancet, 1969; 2: 1229.

was 89 hrs and the individuals had fewer bowl movements compared to the African villagers, where the transit time was only 35 hrs. When the stools were weighed, the weight of the African stools was found to be four times greater than the stools from the British group. These results were not surprising to Dr. Burkitt, as fiber would retain water in the GI tract to increase the stool weight and would reduce the concentration of any possible carcinogens and lower the risk for CRCa. Epidemiological studies have consistently found that diets low in fruit and vegetables increase the risk for CRCa.[189] However, the epidemiological studies analyzing for dietary fiber have provided inconsistent results, and that may be due to the lack of a significant range of fiber intake among U.S. individuals. The recent large European Prospective Investigation into Cancer and Nutrition[190] reported not only an increased risk with consumption of red meat, but a decreased risk with consumption of fiber. Not only does consumption of red meat affect the bile acids, as red meat is generally high in fat, but cooked red meat, especially red meat cooked at very high temperatures, like grilling that results in charring, is associated with the production of heterocyclic aeromatic amines, known carcinogens.

In addition to diet, another lifestyle factor that might aid in reducing the risk for CRCa is regular exercise. The large U.S. Male Health Professionals Study reported that regular exercise (45 min/day) reduced the risk for colon cancer by 50 percent.[191] As the Pritikin Program incorporates all of the epidemiology data related to the CRCa risk, including both diet and exercise, individuals who follow the program should see a dramatically reduced risk for CRCa.

---

[189] Cancer Causes Control, 1991; 2: 427.
[190] Lancet, 2003; 361: 1496.
[191] Annals of Internal Medicine, 1995; 122: 327.

The Pritikin Program and GI Function

In order to evaluate the effects of the Pritikin Program on GI function, a study was undertaken by the American Health Foundation under the direction of Dr. Ernst Wynder. Eleven women from the N.Y. area where the American Health Foundation laboratories were located, who were signed up to attend the Pritikin Program for three weeks, were recruited for the study.[192] Stool samples were collected over 24 hrs for 2 days, weighed and frozen for future analysis of lipids and bile acids. Stool samples were then collected during the final two days of the Pritikin Longevity Center program, weighed, frozen and shipped back to the American Health Foundation laboratory in N.Y. for analysis. Compared to the stool samples collected before the program, after the 3-week Pritikin Program 24-hr. stool weight was increased by 69 percent. Total lipid content of the stools was reduced by 34 percent, total bile acids were reduced by 50 percent and secondary bile acids by 60 percent. These results suggest a major reduction in the risk for CRCa.

---

[192] Preventive Medicine, 1988; 17: 432.

Chapter 6

Obesity and Chronic Inflammation – Risk Factors for Many Health Problems

Since the 1970s obesity has become a worldwide epidemic. For many years the developing countries were almost devoid of obese individuals, but as they adopt a Western lifestyle, obesity is becoming more prevalent. In 1980, 4.8 percent of men and 7.9 percent of women worldwide were considered obese. By 2008 the values had jumped to 9.8 percent for men and 13.8 percent for women with the highest values found in the Westernized countries, including the U.S.[193] At the present time in the United States, two-thirds of adults are overweight, and 32 percent of men and 35 percent of women are considered to be obese. In addition to the obesity problem in U.S. adults is the alarming increase in childhood obesity. In 1980 only 6.5 percent of children aged 6 to 11 years were considered to be obese, but by 2008 the value had increased to nearly 20 percent.[194] For children 2 to 5 years of age, the obesity rate increased from 5 to 10 percent over the same period of time. More alarming is the fact that obesity in 6-month-old infants increased by 73 percent.[195] This increase in childhood obesity is a serious health problem as studies have documented that in more than 80 percent of the cases obese children go on to be obese as adults.[196] Obesity in children increases the number of fat cells in the body, and even with weight loss, the number of cells remains constant and the cells strive to store fat. This is what

---

[193] JAMA, 2012; 307 (5) :483.

[194] Centers for Disease Control and Prevention. NCHS Health EStat: Prevalence of Obesity Among Children and Adolescents: United States, Trends 1963-1965 Through 2007-2008.

[195] Newsweek Magazine, September 21, 2009: "Born to Be Big."

[196] Journal of Adolescent Health, 2008; 42: 512.

makes weight loss so difficult for many obese individuals. Unless people change their lifestyles, the U.S. Government predicts that by 2030 42 percent of the population will be obese.[197] Another major concern is that obesity is now considered to be a state of chronic low-level inflammation and is one of the key factors that makes obesity a risk factor for so many other common health problems.

How is obesity determined?

In large epidemiology or clinical trials, obesity is usually determined according to the body mass index (BMI), which is calculated as the body weight in kilograms divided by the height in meters squared, or in the imperial/English system as weight in pounds times 703 divided by height in inches squared. The web has several sites that do the calculation if you know your height and weight. Here is a good site: (www.cdc.gov/healthyweight/assessing/bmi). A BMI ≥ 25 is considered overweight and a BMI ≥ 30 is considered obese. A person with a BMI below 18.5 is considered to be underweight. Calculating BMI for children and teens up to and including 19 years of age is a bit more complicated as it has to be adjusted for age and sex. The Center for Disease Control and Prevention website has a program to calculate age- and sex-specific BMI and also to give a BMI percentile that gives a relative position for the child's BMI among all children of the same sex and age. A healthy BMI- percentile is within the 5 – 84 percentile, overweight is 85 – 94 percentile, and obese is ≥ 95 percentile.

While the BMI will tell if the body weight is appropriate for the height of the individual, it does *not* tell the amount of body fat, which is the important factor in obesity-related diseases. Some individuals, i.e., weight lifters, might have a BMI of 30 but with a very low percent body fat due to the large amount of muscle mass. More important than the amount of body fat is *where* the fat is

---

[197] American Journal of Preventive Medicine, 2012; 42 (6): 563.

located. Numerous studies have documented that abdominal fat, especially fat in the abdominal cavity also known as visceral fat, fat that has wrapped around inner organs like the stomach, intestines and pancreas is a more serious health risk factor than is subcutaneous (fat under the skin) or lower body fat in the thighs or legs. Waist circumference has been reported to be a most significant risk factor for coronary heart disease and recently has been used as one of the measurements to identify individuals with the metabolic syndrome described in Chapter 4. In a joint scientific statement "Harmonizing the metabolic syndrome"[198] from six international health agencies, it was concluded that the waist measurement cut points for categorizing the metabolic syndrome had to be population- and country-specific. The group from the U.S. representing the American Heart Association and the National Heart Lung and Blood Institute recommended values $\geq$ 40 inches for men and $\geq$ 35 inches for women as the threshold to define abdominal obesity. Other countries used lower values, i.e., $\geq$ 33.5 inches for men and $\geq$ 31.5 inches for women.

How is Body Fat Measured?

The original standard for measuring body fat was hydrostatic or underwater weighing. This technique requires expensive equipment and simply is unacceptable for a lot of individuals, especially the elderly. In view of the problems with hydrostatic weighing, scientists turned to skinfold calipers and developed equations based on measurements at various places around the body. The percent body fat calculated from skinfold fat equations was found to highly correlate with the results obtained from hydrostatic weighing, at least in younger individuals. Thus, for many years skinfold calipers were used in many programs and are still used today in some sports clubs and by personal trainers. The development of new equipment such as bioelectrical

---

[198] Circulation, 2009; 120: 1640.

impedance and dual-energy x-ray absorptiometry (DEXA) has made the assessment of body fat simple. DEXA is the method presently used at the Pritikin Longevity Center. DEXA is a scan technique where the individual lies on a table, and the entire body is scanned with low energy x-ray. It takes 15 – 30 minutes, depending on the size of the individual, to complete the scan. In addition to measuring body fat, including abdominal fat, DEXA can also be used to measure bone density to detect osteoporosis. A healthy body fat for males should be in the range of 14 – 17 percent of body weight, and for females in the range of 21 – 24 percent. Some male athletes, however, may have values as low as 5 percent. Once the percent body fat is known, it can be used to give the individual his or her ideal body weight.

But each patient requires individual attention. Giving an individual an ideal body weight may be okay for the individual who is 10 – 15 pounds overweight, but telling a 300-pound man that his ideal body weight is 180 pounds may be counterproductive. In this individual, who already knows he is grossly overweight, the focus should *not* be an ideal body weight; rather, the focus should be on risk factors such as blood pressure, diabetes, cholesterol, triglycerides, etc., because excessively overweight/obese individuals might see dramatic improvements in these risk factors in a very short period of time, and with only a small weight loss as has been documented at the Pritikin Program. Focusing on these factors would give obese individuals more incentive to continue with the program, whereas if they focus solely on an ideal body weight, which they may never achieve, they may get discouraged and abandon the healthy lifestyle. For the past 30 years at the Pritikin Longevity Center, the faculty has seen how motivating improvements in risk factors like cholesterol and blood pressure can be. People who walk into Pritikin obsessed with their excess weight leave Pritikin realizing that success encompasses *much more* than what the bathroom scale says.

They're thrilled at the health results they've achieved, and they're jubilantly announcing to everyone they see: "You won't believe how much my cholesterol went down," or "The last time my blood pressure was this low I was in high school," or "I never thought I could feel this good again." Best of all, they're motivated, like never before, to continue with their healthy new habits when they return home. They've learned that while weight loss is slow, getting healthy can happen very, very quickly.

While many techniques can measure total body fat, they cannot measure the amount of abdominal fat. DEXA does measure fat in the abdominal region, combined subcutaneous and intra-abdominal. The only accurate way to measure only the intra-abdominal or visceral fat is with MRI or CT scans done only in hospital or clinical settings. MRI or CT scans have been used in some experimental studies but would not be done otherwise just to measure body fat.

If you don't have access to any of these methods of measuring body fat, there are a few simple tests you might use. First, ask yourself, what is your weight today compared to what it was when you graduated from high school or college? If it is the same or more, you have more than likely gained body fat because as we age we tend to lose muscle mass as we become less physically active. A second simple test is to take off all of your clothes and stand in front of a mirror. If you look fat, you *are* fat and need to lose weight (or gain a lot of muscle). A third test is to pinch the skin on the back of your hand. This is generally two pieces of skin with no fat. Now pinch yourself at different places and see if the pinch is thicker. A pinch thicker than the back of your hand is due primarily to subcutaneous fat.

What Causes Obesity?

As explained in Chapter 1, obesity can be explained by the first law of thermodynamics: calories in = calories out ± calories stored. In quick summary, this equation means that energy (the scientific word for calories) is not created or destroyed, only transformed. Calories consumed in food or drink must be burned or stored. Any excess calories are stored in the body as fat. Since the 1970s, when the obesity epidemic was just starting, until the present time, average calorie intake in the U.S. has increased from 2450 to 2618 calories per day for men and from 1542 to 1877 calories per day for women (one pound of body weight equals 3500 calories).[199] Fat consumption has changed little, despite all the emphasis on low-fat foods. Refined sugar consumption, most particularly high fructose corn syrup, has contributed to most of the excess calories. The availability of excess calories is due in large part to the "super-size" concept generated by the food industry, especially the fast-food industry, as well as the availability of calorie-rich foods with little satiety, or stomach-filling, impact, i.e., high-fat foods. On the other side of the equation is the fact that individuals have become more sedentary as they spend more time watching TV and working or playing at computers.

Unfortunately, obesity cannot be explained simply on the basis of the first law of thermodynamics. While no one can argue the importance of the first law to explain obesity, *how* different individuals respond to the first law depends on genes, hormones, the type of foods consumed, and possibly exposure to certain chemicals. We all know of individuals who seem to eat constantly and never gain weight. Conversely, some individuals seem to eat very little and still gain weight. Several studies have confirmed that when individuals are overfed calories, there is a significant difference in weight gain. In classic studies of identical twins, Dr. Claude Bouchard and colleagues demonstrated a genetic basis for the range of responses to either overfeeding (positive energy

---

[199] U.S. Department of Agriculture. U.S. food supply: nutrients and other food components, 1970 to 2000. Economic Research Service; 2001. Available on-line at http://www.ers.usda.gov/data/foodconsumption/NutrientAvailIndex.htm.

balance) or increased exercise (negative energy balance).[200] Twelve pairs of young male identical twins were overfed 1,000 calories a day, 6 days per week, over a 100-day period. The average weight gain was 18 pounds with a range of 9 to 29 pounds. When one twin gained a lot of weight, so did the other, indicating a genetic influence. In the study, the subjects experienced a small gain in fat-free mass, i.e., muscle, while most of the weight gain was in fat. The increases in total body fat did not predict increases in visceral fat, indicating a genetic influence as to *where* excess calories are deposited.

Several studies have also found that spot reducing does not work other than liposuction. In other words, you cannot exercise one specific part of the body and expect to lose body fat in that area. So don't be swayed by those late-night infomercials promising 6-pack abs from a machine that works solely on your stomach muscles. It won't help *unless* you're supplementing these ab workouts with a healthy eating plan like Pritikin and daily aerobic exercise, such as walking or running.

For the negative energy balance experiment (the exercise portion), Dr. Bouchard and colleagues studied seven pairs of identical twins over a period of 93 days.[201] The subjects were exercised twice a day (9 out of 10 days) on an exercycle. After three months, the average weight loss was 11 pounds. Again, there was a large variation in the amount of weight loss, and again there was good agreement within twin pairs. All of the weight loss was in body fat with a striking amount of intra-abdominal fat loss. At the end of the three-month training period, while exercising at the same submaximal workload, the subjects burned more fat calories compared to carbohydrate calories than they did at the start of the study. This study also confirms a genetic aspect to weight control and also demonstrates that exercise can be important for weight

---

[200] New England Journal of Medicine, 1990; 322: 1477.
[201] Obesity, 1994; 2 (5): 400.

loss, but by itself is rather inefficient in the sense that it takes a lot of work over the course of months to achieve a significant weight loss. However, it does point out the importance of exercise for burning excess body fat, especially abdominal fat.

Hormones, including insulin, cortisol, thyroxin and estrogen, can also influence body metabolism and fat deposition. Insulin, the hormone described in Chapter 4 as a primary factor responsible for moving glucose (sugar) from the bloodstream into body cells, also regulates the movement of fats (fatty acids) from the bloodstream into body cells, mainly fat and muscle cells. Insulin regulates the clearance of fats from the blood by activating an enzyme, lipoprotein lipase (LPL). LPL is produced in fat and muscle cells and moves to the capillary wall where it attacks fat particles (chylomicrons or triglycerides) when they float by and removes fatty acids. In muscle, these fatty acids can be used for fuel during exercise. Some excess fatty acid can also be stored in muscle cells. In fat cells, the fatty acids are stored as excess energy (triglycerides) until they are called on to be used as fuel for exercise. Insulin, which is elevated in insulin resistant or type 2 diabetic individuals, suppresses LPL activity in muscle and activates it in fat cells, resulting in increased fat deposition. And sure enough, it is well known that when type 2 diabetics start on insulin they invariably gain weight/fat. In the exercise experiment described earlier on twins, one of the reasons they were burning more fat calories relative to carbohydrate calories during exercise at the end of the study was likely due to increased LPL activity in muscle as well as lower insulin levels.

Another hormone that plays a role in regulating both glucose and fat metabolism is cortisol. Cortisol, also known as the "stress hormone," is released from the adrenal gland in response to physical, mental or emotional stress. Physical stress, i.e., exercise, increases cortisol secretion that impacts several physiological functions. It increases blood levels of glucose and free fatty acids to be used as fuel by the active muscles, and it increases heart rate and blood pressure to aid in performance. Following exercise, blood levels of cortisol fall back to normal low levels. Conversely, chronic mental or emotional stress can result in constant elevations in cortisol, and the elevated cortisol responses have negative long-term impacts on the body. In addition, prolonged elevation of cortisol can result in increased appetite, resulting in "emotional eating," leading to visceral obesity. One of the best ways to relieve the chronic stress response is regular aerobic exercise. Activities such as yoga and Tai Chi can also be effective ways of reducing stress.

Thyroxin, a hormone released from the thyroid gland located in the neck, is involved in controlling the rate of metabolism in the body as well as influencing physical development. It has been estimated that more than 20 percent of those over the age of 65 years suffer from hypothyroidism (low thyroxin). Hypothyroidism is far more common in women compared to men. Individuals with hypothyroidism have a low basal rate of metabolism, elevated cholesterol, and may suffer from depression and chronic fatigue. The exact cause(s) of hypothyroidism are unknown. These people are usually, but not always, overweight/obese with increased abdominal obesity. Thyroid medication may in fact help correct hypothyroidism, so if you have any of the above symptoms you should see your doctor for more information and diagnostic testing.

Estrogen is another hormone that affects fat deposition. It is well known that women have more body fat than men. Women generally have their fat in the hips, thighs, and buttocks (pear shape) compared to the abdominal fat (apple shape) generally seen in men. Using isolated fat samples obtained at the time of surgery, scientists have confirmed that estrogen stimulates proliferation of preadipocytes (fat cells without any stored fat) in both men and women.[202] Preadipocytes from women were more responsive to estrogen than preadipocytes from men. When the number of preadipocytes increases, so does the body's ability to store fat. One of the unexplained aspects of estrogen and obesity has been why women generally gain weight after menopause when estrogen levels are very low. The answer may lie in experimental studies reported at a recent American Chemical Society meeting. Scientists found that estrogen receptors in the brain area known as the hypothalamus regulate food intake (satiety) and metabolism and are activated by estrogen to reduce appetite and food intake and to increase metabolism. When the estrogen receptors in the female brains were blocked in animals, they immediately began to eat more food, burn less energy, and pack on the excess calories as fat, especially in the abdominal region. This indicates that postmenopausal women have to pay special attention to what they eat and how much exercise they do on a daily basis so they don't pack the excess calories into existing fat cells.

In 2002 an unknown scientist by the name of Paula Baillie-Hamilton published an article in the *Journal of Alternative and Complementary Medicine* suggesting that the obesity epidemic was related to the explosion in the number of man-made chemicals introduced into our environment since the 1970s, many with estrogenic effects.[203] At the present time, there are over 80,000 man-made chemicals approved for use in the U.S. with no clue as to the impact they have on human health. In 2009 (Sept. 21) an article appeared in *Newsweek* "Born to be Big" providing evidence that early exposure to common chemicals may be programming kids to be fat. Here is some of the evidence:

---

[202] The Journal of Clinical Endocrinology & Metabolism, 2001; 86: 5045.
[203] Journal of Alternative and Complementary Medicine, 2002; 8 (2): 185.

- A 73 percent increase in the number of obese (> 95 percentile body weight) 6-month-old babies has been observed since 1970,
- Stem cells exposed to chemicals turn into fat cells,
- Mice exposed to estrogen/chemicals during pregnancy are born with more fat cells,
- Some commonly used pesticides have estrogenic effects and have been shown to increase the risk for obesity.

The type of foods consumed can also have an important impact on fat accumulation in the body. As pointed out in Chapter 1, fat contains 9 calories per gram while carbohydrates and protein each only contain 4 calories per gram. Thus, eating high-fat foods increases calorie intake, especially since they have the lowest satiety, or hunger-curbing, factor, resulting in overeating. In addition, fat is more easily stored as it can be directly deposited into fat cells, while carbohydrates and protein have to be converted to fat before storage in fat cells, a process that burns calories.

In earlier chapters, I described experiments on rodents placed on a high-fat refined-sugar/refined-carbohydrate diet (typical U.S. diet) compared to a low-fat starch/unrefined carbohydrate diet (similar to Pritikin). The HFS rodents became insulin resistant with hyperinsulinemia and developed the metabolic syndrome. The animals also gained weight and abdominal fat. The interesting observation was that the HFS animals realized that their diet was packed with calories due to the high-caloric density of the food and actually consumed less food compared to the low-fat diet group. When the food intake was measured and the calorie consumption calculated, there was no difference in calorie intake between the two groups, despite the fact that the HFS group gained weight and got fat. This study clearly demonstrates the importance of paying attention to the *kind* of foods consumed and not just the calories. In other words, just counting calories is not the best way to lose excess weight or excess fat and be healthy. Our research may also help explain why so many Americans who do work hard trying to lose weight – judiciously counting calories, and eating just half of their typical portions of burgers, fries, and potato chips – net so little in return. They often fail and, understandably so, become discouraged and quit. On the flip side, our research may also explain why many people attending the Pritikin Longevity Center are surprised at *how much* they can eat, far more than those meager servings of burgers and chips, yet successfully shed weight. Bottom Line: You can eat *more* and weigh *less* when you're eating the *right* foods – water-rich, nutrient-rich, fiber-rich whole foods like fruits, vegetables, beans, and starchy vegetables like yams, corn, and potatoes.

Impact of the Pritikin Program on Body Weight

In keeping with the first law of thermodynamics, it should not be surprising that individuals adopting the Pritikin lifestyle should lose weight due to the low calorie density of the low-fat, high-complex-carbohydrate diet combined with the daily exercise. In the study of 4587 adults who attended the Pritikin 3-week residential program, the males lost an average of 12.1 lbs. (5.5 Kg) and the females an average of 7.2 lbs. (3.3 Kg).[204] During a 2-week stay at the Pritikin Center, overweight/obese children age 10-17 yrs. lost an average of 8.8 lbs (4 Kg) and reduced their waist circumference by 4.8 percent.[205] In the 5-year follow-up study of 64 CAD patients discussed in Chapter 2, body weight was reduced from 174 lbs. to 163 lbs in 3 weeks at the Center, and at follow-up was reported to be 163 lbs.[206] In the 2-3 year follow-up study of 69 type 2 diabetic patients discussed in Chapter 4, body weight was

---

[204] Archives of Internal Medicine, 1991; 151: 1389.
[205] Metabolism Clinical and Experimental, 2006; 55: 871.
[206] Journal of Cardiac Rehabilitation, 1983; 3: 183.

reduced from 172 lbs. to 162 lbs. while at the Center for three weeks and at follow-up was reported to be 158 lbs.[207] Thus, it is evident that the Pritikin lifestyle is important for weight control – not only shedding excess weight but keeping it off long-term. More importantly is the impact the Pritikin Program has on fat cell function, to be discussed shortly.

Pritikin Weight Loss Secret

There is no secret as to why the Pritikin Program leads to weight loss. In keeping with the first law of thermodynamics previously discussed, the Pritikin Program works on both sides of the equation by increasing caloric expenditure via daily exercise and reducing calorie intake by following the Pritikin Eating Plan guidelines. The Pritikin Eating Plan is low in calories due to the low-fat content and the fact that just about all of the fruits, vegetables and whole grains are very low in calorie density due to their high-water and high-fiber content. This combination of increased calorie expenditure and low-calorie density foods allows one to eat five or six meals and snacks daily, to feel satiated, and still lose weight and keep it off. Remember that losing weight is not the primary goal; changing lifestyle is. You did not gain all of the excess weight overnight, so don't expect to lose it overnight – but it will come off! In the following sections it will become clear why focusing on changing lifestyle is far more important than focusing on losing weight for overall health.

Fat Cells – More Than Calorie Banks

For many years, the only function of fat cells scientists knew about was that fat cells were the holding places where excess calories ended up. Fatty acids were removed from the circulation through the action of the enzyme LPL (previously described) and converted into triglycerides for storage. With exercise or negative

---

[207] Diabetes Care, 1983; 6: 268.

caloric balance, another enzyme in the fat cells, hormone-sensitive lipase, would be activated to degrade the stored triglycerides and release free fatty acids into the circulation to be used by muscle as fuel. In 1950 a protein named leptin was found to be produced in fat cells and was shown to depress appetite and increase metabolism in mice. Mice born with a genetic defect and did not produce leptin were found to be voracious eaters, had low metabolism, and became obese.

The discovery of leptin and the fact that it was shown to regulate appetite and metabolism via activation of receptors in the brains of mice was initially heralded as a major breakthrough and was thought to be the answer to controlling obesity by using leptin pills to curb appetite and increase metabolism. Strangely, several studies reported that serum levels of leptin were directly correlated with the extent of obesity in humans. So why do obese humans have elevated levels of leptin if it is supposed to curb appetite and increase metabolism? The clinical trials with obese individuals given leptin were a major disappointment as it was discovered that obese individuals are resistant to the action of leptin in the brain centers that control food intake and metabolism. Thus, the subjects did not lose weight in spite of elevated levels of serum leptin. There was more troubling news. Other functions attributed to the actions of leptin were discovered, including activation of the sympathetic nervous system to increase blood pressure, which explains in part why obesity is an important risk factor for hypertension. Other factors associated with the development of atherosclerosis were found to be increased by leptin. Fortunately, research done on Pritikin Program participants has shown that serum levels of leptin are dramatically reduced in just a few weeks, and with only minimal weight loss.[208] Although obese individuals generally have more fat cells capable of producing leptin, the

[208] American Journal of Physiology: Endocrinology & Metabolism, 2012; 303: E542.

Pritikin results indicate that something in the body responsive to a healthy lifestyle regulates the leptin production.

Following the discovery that leptin was produced by fat cells, the molecular biologists soon demonstrated that fat cells produced a host of proteins, more than fifty to date, that impact various body functions. Another important protein found to be produced by fat cells is adiponectin. Unlike leptin, whose serum levels directly correlate with body fat, adiponectin is inversely correlated with the extent of body fat. In other words, more body fat is associated with *reduced* adiponectin production by fat cells. The reduction in serum levels of adiponectin is bad as adiponectin is known to have many positive effects. Higher levels of adiponectin have been found to increase fat metabolism, reduce triglycerides, decrease inflammatory factors, increase insulin sensitivity, and reduce production of cell adhesion molecules related to atherosclerosis development.

Other important proteins produced in fat cells are inflammatory cytokines. They're important because their actions provide a link between obesity and many of the common health problems associated with obesity.

Obesity and Inflammation

Inflammation is a normal response in the body when it is under attack by foreign invaders like bacteria, virus, or cancer cells and is characterized by redness, heat, pain, and swelling at the sight of infection. These symptoms are triggered by white blood cells, which have "rushed" to the sight and release chemicals known as inflammatory cytokines. White blood cells make up the body's immune system and accumulate at the site where the body is invaded by bacteria or virus.

Monocytes (one of the types of white blood cells) are the first responders and play an important role in the development of inflammation due to their ability to produce and release large amounts of inflammatory cytokines. Monocytes are produced in the bone marrow and then released into the circulation. Some of the monocytes immediately leave the circulation and enter tissues where they act as "housekeepers" by cleaning up dead debris and releasing anti-inflammatory cytokines (i.e.IL-10) to maintain a healthy environment for normal cell function.

The monocyte membranes contain Toll-Like Receptors (TLRs) that have the ability to detect foreign invaders like bacteria and viruses. Think of TLRs as the "security systems" for your body. When they detect trouble, they sound "alarms." There are eleven different TLRs on the monocyte membranes of humans that have the ability to detect a wide array of bacteria or virus. When the monocyte TLRs are activated, they in turn activate Nuclear Factor kappa B (NFkB) (see Figure 6.1) allowing it to enter the nucleus and activate the genes responsible for producing other related factors that attempt to destroy the foreign invaders. Think of NFkB as the final "power switch" that "turns on" the production of pro-inflammatory cytokine genes. Not only does the activated monocyte produce the pro-inflammatory cytokines, it also produces MCP-1, a protein that attracts more monocytes from the circulation to the infected area, resulting in a major inflammatory response. This function of monocytes is obviously important for protecting the body from foreign invaders. Not only do monocytes enter tissues infected with bacteria or virus, they also enter adipose (fat) tissue where they create a state of chronic low-level inflammation with a constant release of inflammatory cytokines. In previous chapters the role of inflammation in the initiation and development of many common diseases (coronary disease, type 2 diabetes, cancers) was discussed as well as the fact that pro-inflammatory cytokines and obesity were major risk

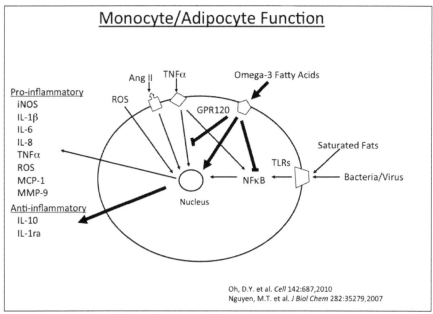

Monocyte/Adipocyte Function

Pro-inflammatory
iNOS
IL-1β
IL-6
IL-8
TNFα
ROS
MCP-1
MMP-9

Anti-inflammatory
IL-10
IL-1ra

Ang II TNFα   Omega-3 Fatty Acids

ROS

GPR120

Saturated Fats

TLRs

NFκB

Bacteria/Virus

Nucleus

Oh, D.Y. et al. *Cell* 142:687,2010
Nguyen, M.T. et al. *J Biol Chem* 282:35279,2007

Figure 6.1 Functions of monocytes and fat cells. The thin lines depict factors involved in the production of pro-inflammatory factors while the thicker lines depict factors that block pro-inflammatory pathways and activate anti-inflammatory pathways. Oh, D.Y et al. *Cell* 142:687, 2010. Nguyen, M. T. et al. *J Biol Chem* 282:35279, 2007.

factors. Chronic low-level inflammation is thought to be one of the major factors linking obesity to various diseases. For example, C-Reactive Protein, a marker for inflammation, was discussed in Chapter 2 as a risk factor for atherosclerosis and heart attacks. Chronic low levels of CRP indicative of chronic low-grade inflammation are of concern and are referred to as hs-CRP (high-sensitivity CRP) as it takes a special assay to measure the very low levels. According to the American Heart Association, serum levels of hs-CRP lower than 1.0 mg/L are low risk for atherosclerosis, 1-3 mg/L is average risk and higher than 3.0 is high risk. A value higher than 10 mg/L indicates systemic infection, caused by a flu virus, staph infection, or other invasions, and the test needs to be repeated at a later date after the infection is treated. However, not all research supports the importance of serum hsCRP as a good predictor of heart attacks.

For many years it was thought that only white blood cells contained the NFkB "power switch" and genes that had the ability to generate the production of inflammatory cytokines. However, more recently it has been demonstrated that many other tissues, including fat cells, contain TRLs and the NFkB switch. So what turns on the NFkB switch in the absence of bacteria or virus? Exciting research by Dr. Jerrold Olefsky and colleagues at U.C. San Diego reported in 2007 that when mice were placed on a high-saturated-fat diet, there was an invasion of monocytes into the adipose tissues and inflammatory cytokine levels increased in the circulation.[209] The mice also became insulin resistant. Chronic insulin resistance could eventually lead to type 2 diabetes, as discussed in Chapter 4. The increase in inflammatory cytokines was due to activation of the NFkB switch by TLRs in response to saturated fats in both monocytes and fat cells, as shown in Figure 6.1. When Olefsky's group added omega-3 fatty acids to the high-fat diet, they blocked the production of pro-inflammatory cytokines and increased the production of anti-inflammatory factors, as shown in Figure 6.1, thus documenting the value of consuming fish to reduce low-level inflammation. Research at Cornell Cancer Center has recently shown that high-fat diets increased inflammatory factors that increased aromatase activity in fat cells,[210] which in turn increases estrogen levels in females, linking high-fat diets to an increased risk of breast cancer.

Another tissue that is known to contain the NFkB power switch and the ability to produce pro-inflammatory cytokines and related factors is the endothelium that lines the artery wall and plays an important role in the development of atherosclerosis, as discussed in Chapter 2. As endothelial cells also contain TLRs,

---

[209] Annual Review of Physiology, 2010; 72: 219.
[210] Cancer Prevention Research, 2011; 4: 329.

they can respond to high-saturated-fat diets to turn on the NFkB switch, produce pro-inflammatory cytokines, generate ROS to oxidize LDL, and produce MCP-1 to attract monocytes into the artery wall, all factors involved in the development of atherosclerosis. So not only do high-saturated-fat diets increase serum cholesterol, as discussed in Chapter 2, they basically induce the whole atherosclerotic process.

This same type of high-fat diet, through activation of the NFkB power switch, increases production of matrix metalloproteinase (MMP) enzymes that lead to erosion of connective tissues. MMP-9 has been shown to be involved in rupture of the fibrous cap covering the cholesterol plaque, resulting in a heart attack or stroke. MMP-1, along with high concentrations of monocytes, has also been reported to be elevated in the joints of patients with arthritis.

Tumor tissue has also been found to contain the NFkB power switch and produce inflammatory cytokines. But unlike other tissues, where inflammatory cytokines try to destroy the foreign invaders, in tumor tissue the inflammatory cytokines *stimulate* cancer cell growth and block apoptosis (cancer cell death). Cancerous tissues attract monocytes and so, as in fat tissue, there is interaction between NFkB in the tissues and the monocytes in that NFkB powers up the monocytes' production of inflammatory cytokines and increases ROS generation to stimulate tumor growth.

More recently, it has been reported that skeletal muscle contains TLRs and the NFkB pathway.[211] Thus, NFkB production of pro-inflammatory factors in response to high-saturated fat diets may be involved in the observed insulin resistance as reported by Olefsky's group. When inflammatory factors rise, it appears that the muscle cells' resistance to insulin action also rises, which

---

[211] Cell, 2004; 119: 285.

means that anything causing the escalation of inflammatory factors, such as the saturated-fat diets observed by Olefsy's group, could well be contributing to the development of insulin resistance and eventually type 2 diabetes. Activation of the NFkB pathway releasing pro-inflammatory cytokines may be involved in the loss of muscle mass and strength (sarcopenia) commonly associated with aging. The loss of both muscle mass and strength with aging can be prevented to a great extent through resistance training. Of course, reducing the saturated fat while increasing the omega-3 fat content of the diet to reduce activation of the NFkB pathway would also be important.

Effects of the Pritikin Program on Inflammatory Factors

In Chapter 2 it was stated that the Pritikin Program has been reported to substantially reduce (up to 45 percent) serum levels of hs-CRP,[212] a general marker of inflammation in men, women and children. CRP is produced primarily by the liver and released into the circulation when levels of inflammatory cytokines, i.e. TNFα, are increased. Thus, we obtained serum samples from overweight/obese children attending the Pritikin Program to measure levels of inflammatory factors. After just two weeks of the diet and exercise program, serum levels of pro-inflammatory cytokines were reduced significantly. TNFα was reduced by 43 percent, IL-6 by 56 percent and IL-8 by 30 percent.[213] Similar results have also been obtained from adults attending the Pritikin Program.

To further test the effects of the Pritikin Program on the production of inflammatory cytokines, cell culture tests were conducted using serum from participants. Tests were conducted with serum-stimulated fat cell and monocyte cultures before and

---

[212] Metabolism, 2004; 53: 377. Journal of Applied Physiology, 2006; 100: 1657. Atherosclerosis, 2007; 191: 98.
[213] American Journal of Physiology: Endocrinology & Metabolism, 2012; 303: E542.

after the Pritikin Program. When the cytokines secreted by the fat cell and the monocytes cultures were measured, the production of pro-inflammatory cytokines was reduced after the Pritikin Program.[214] This reduction in pro-inflammatory cytokines was observed in just two weeks, and with little weight loss, in other words, while the subjects remained overweight or obese. These results support the previous statement regarding the importance of a healthy lifestyle over a focus on weight loss, per se. The good news is that the Pritikin Program has been documented to achieve both: better health within just two to three weeks, plus a leaner, fitter body in the weeks, months, and years that follow.

As previously stated, inflammatory cytokines and the NFkB pathway are found in tumor cells where they stimulate growth and block apoptosis of the tumor cells. Using our prostate cancer cell culture methods discussed in Chapter 5, we measured activation of the NFkB pathway following serum stimulation of prostate cancer cells. In the serum samples from men who had been following the Pritikin Program for two weeks, there was far less NFkB activation in the cancer cells as well as reduced tumor cell growth and increased apoptosis compared to pre-Pritikin serum samples from the men.[215] These results emphasize the importance of following the Pritikin Program for individuals diagnosed with prostate cancer, and probably for other forms of cancer, where inflammation is involved, as discussed in Chapter 5.

Additional tests were run on serum samples from overweight/obese subjects to measure other fat cell factors, including leptin and adiponectin. Leptin was reduced by over 50 percent while adiponectin was increased by 35 percent – both

---

[214] American Journal of Physiology: Endocrinology & Metabolism, 2012; 303: E542.
[215] eCAM, 2011; 2011: ID 529053, 1-7.

excellent outcomes.[216] These changes in leptin and adiponectin are important as leptin is positively correlated with coronary disease while adiponectin is inversely correlated with coronary disease, meaning, the *higher* your levels of leptin, the greater your risk of coronary disease, and the *lower* your levels of adiponectin, the greater your risk of the disease. In other studies related to heart disease, we also reported reductions in serum MCP-1, PAI-1 and MMP-9 following the Pritikin Program,[217] and these reductions may have reflected changes in fat cell and/or monocyte function.

What aspects of the Pritikin Program might be important in reducing the pro-inflammatory factors? Probably the most important is the dramatic reduction in the consumption of saturated fat because this dietary change alone would dramatically reduce chronic activation of the TLRs and NFkB pathways involved in the production of pro-inflammatory factors. In recent studies of adults attending the Pritikin Program, we documented a 20 – 30 percent reduction is serum saturated fatty acids,[218] and in children the reduction was as high as 40 percent.[219] The consumption of cold-water fish three times each week would also increase the levels of omega-3 fatty acids, which would further reduce the levels of pro-inflammatory cytokines, as shown in Figure 6.1. In addition to the dramatic reduction in dietary saturated fat (to < 4 percent of calories), the reduction in total fat (to < 15 percent of calories) and the replacement of refined sugars with complex carbohydrates would reduce the formation of ROS that can also stimulate the production of pro-inflammatory factors (see Figure 6.1). In Chapter 2, I described experiments done on endothelial cell cultures stimulated with serum and showed that serum obtained

---

[216] American Journal of Physiology: Endocrinology & Metabolism, 2012; 303: E542.
[217] Journal of Applied Physiology, 2006; 100: 1657.
[218] Unpublished data.
[219] American Journal of Physiology: Endocrinology & Metabolism, 2012; 303: E542.

from subjects after the Pritikin Program substantially reduced ROS formation. Along this same line is the importance of regular exercise, which has been shown to increase anti-oxidant enzymes in the body to reduce ROS levels.

Thus, it should be obvious from this discussion that obesity and inflammation are related factors and explain, in part, why obesity is a well-known risk factor for so many different health problems. It should also be obvious that adopting the Pritikin lifestyle is far more important than focusing on weight loss, per se, to prevent and/or control many of the common health problems seen in the industrialized world and now appearing in the developing countries. Simply cutting calories and not focusing on dramatically reducing the consumption of saturated fats would be less effective for reducing chronic inflammation and the risk for related health problems. Bottom Line: All of us want not only a lean body but a healthy one. The Pritikin Program can provide both.

Chapter 7

Dementia and Alzheimer's

As people get older, they generally experience some forgetfulness such as recalling names, dates, etc. This is termed mild cognitive impairment and is associated with a decrease in brain size seen in older individuals but is thought to be a normal part of aging. While this mild cognitive impairment may be common in the industrialized areas of the world, in his book *Healthy at 100* John Robbins reported that not only were the centenarians living in non-industrialized areas of the world healthy and free from common Western diseases, they were also mentally alert. A few studies with older Americans have shown that adopting a regular exercise program can improve cognitive function even in patients with Alzheimer's.[220] These improvements have been correlated with improved blood flow to the brain with regular exercise. Other studies have reported that older individuals who undergo mental challenges on a regular basis, such as crossword puzzles, show improved cognitive function.[221]

Studies with animals have reported that aging is associated with a decrease in brain levels of a protein known as brain-derived neurotrophic factor (BDNF), especially in the area of the brain known as the hippocampus.[222] BDNF is a growth factor found in the brains of both humans and rodents that supports the survival of existing neurons (nerve cells), and encourages the growth and differentiation of new neurons and synapses (nerve connections); thus, BDNF is important for

---

[220] Journal of Nursing Scholarship, 2006; 38(4): 358.
[221] Journal of Preventive Medicine and Public Health, 2013; 46 (1): S22. doi: 10.3961/jpmph.2013.46.S.S22. Epub 2013 Jan 30.
[222] Brain Research Reviews, 2008; 59 (1): 201.

cognition and long-term memory. We conducted research with Dr. Fernando Gomez-Pinilla, a neurobiochemist at UCLA, to study brain-derived neurotrophic factor (BDNF) in our rodent model of diet-induced metabolic syndrome (Chapter 4). When our rodents were raised on the high-fat, refined-sugar (HFS) diet (similar to the typical Western diet), BDNF levels in the brain were reduced and cognitive function (learning) in the Morris Swimming Maze was impaired compared to animals raised on a low-fat, starch diet (similar to the Pritikin Eating Plan).[223] If the animals were given access to running wheels for daily exercise while on the HFS diet, the reductions in BDNF and cognitive function were prevented. Not surprising were the results obtained on the rodents raised on the low-fat, complex-carbohydrate diet given daily exercise (Pritikin Program); they had the highest levels of BDNF and the best performance in the swim maze. In more recent studies Dr. Gomez-Pinilla and his group reported that supplementing the low-fat, complex-carbohydrate diet with the omega-3 fatty acid DHA increased the brain content of BDNF by approximately 25 percent and enhanced performance in the swim maze by the same amount.[224] When they added exercise to the DHA-supplemented group, both brain BDNF levels and learning were increased by almost 50 percent.[225] It is results like these, as well as other scientific evidence, that led to the Pritikin Program adding wild cold-water fish to the diet several days a week to enhance the intake of omega-3 fatty acids. Adopting the Pritikin Program including the diet, low in fat (especially saturated fat) and increased omega-3 fats, combined with daily exercise should enhance long-term memory and cognitive function. Whether or not the Pritikin Program can prevent Alzheimer's is unknown.

---

[223] Neuroscience, 2002; 112: 803.
[224] Nature Reviews Neuroscience, 2008; 9 (7): 568.
[225] Neuroscience, 2008; 155 (3): 751.

When declines in mental functions such as memory, thinking, and reasoning become severe enough to interfere with daily functioning, the individual is suffering from true dementia and a significant loss of brain cells. Unfortunately, the loss of brain cells starts well before the onset of signs of dementia. Once dementia is diagnosed, it is usually progressive and can only be reversed in a small percentage (< 20 percent) of cases.[226] Substance abuse (drugs or alcohol) has been reported to be associated with dementia that was reversed when the abuse was stopped. Some medications have also been reported to be associated with dementia that was improved when the medications were stopped. Dementia has also been reported in patients following heart surgery where the patients were placed on a heart-lung machine for extended periods. There are at least 50 known causes of classical dementia, but by far the most common causes accounting for 80-90 percent of all dementia in the U.S. are Alzheimer's and vascular dementia. These two causes of dementia are often found in the same individual.

Vascular dementia results from conditions that damage the brain's blood vessels, reducing their ability to deliver the needed oxygen and nutrients to the brain cells to support their normal functions. A lack of oxygen and nutrients results not only in a loss of brain cell function but eventually brain cell death. A stroke may or may not lead to dementia depending on the specific area of the brain affected. There are two main kinds of stroke, ischemic and hemorrhagic (bleeding). An ischemic stroke is the result of atherosclerosis developing in a large artery that supplies the brain. This is described in detail in Chapter 2. When the atherosclerotic cholesterol plaque ruptures, a clot forms and blocks blood flow and oxygen delivery to a specific area of the brain, resulting in a stroke. This is the most common cause of stroke in the U.S., and if dementia occurs suddenly, it is referred

---

[226] Journal of Neurology, 1995; 242 (7): 466.

to as "post-stroke dementia." A hemorrhagic stroke occurs when a vessel in the brain suddenly ruptures. Dementia may also develop suddenly following a hemorrhagic stroke if the rupture results in a massive leakage of blood into the brain. Vascular dementia can also develop gradually as a result of a series of "mini strokes" resulting from small blood vessel damage caused by severe hypertension, diabetes, or inflammatory conditions known to damage small blood vessels. Diabetes is especially known to damage small blood vessels in other tissues, including the kidney and eye. Vascular dementia can also develop following brain injury sustained in concussions. This type of dementia may be seen in professional athletes involved in contact sports such as football or boxing, or in soldiers exposed to explosive devices.

The most common cause of dementia in the U.S. is Alzheimer's disease, responsible for 50-80 percent of all dementia. A recent National Institutes of Health report (2010) concluded that the cause of Alzheimer's is unknown, but there are some signs that the risk for Alzheimer's is increased with diabetes, high cholesterol and smoking.[227] These three things are all lifestyle related and suggest that Alzheimer's might be prevented with proper lifestyle change. Further evidence for the involvement of lifestyle in the development of Alzheimer's is the fact that there has been a significant increase in the incidence of Alzheimer's in the past 15-20 years. Part of the increased incidence may be due to increased recognition of symptoms leading to increased diagnoses. However, between 2000-2008, when mortality from major diseases including heart disease, stroke, prostate and breast cancers was dropping in the U.S., death from Alzheimer's increased by 66 percent.[228] It is now the

---

[227] http://www.nia.nih.gov/sites/default/files/2010_alzheimers_disease_ progress_report_.pdf
[228] http://www.alz.org/documents_custom/2011_facts_figures_fact_sheet.pdf

sixth leading cause of death in the U.S. People, in effect, may be dying in fewer numbers from *some* cardiovascular-related conditions, like heart disease, but deaths from *other* potentially cardiovascular-related conditions, particularly Alzheimer's, are increasing.

What is well established regarding Alzheimer's is the presence in the brain of deposits of amyloid protein as well as another protein called tau, as detected at autopsy. Whether these deposits are the cause or simply a marker for Alzheimer's is not established at this time. A recent study funded by the National Institute on Aging examined 159 volunteers age 51 to 88 who started the study with no signs of cognitive impairment and were followed over time. Using brain scans, amyloid deposits were quantitated and cognitive function was assessed. Over time, 23 participants developed mild cognitive impairment and 9 were eventually diagnosed with Alzheimer's disease. The 9 subjects who developed Alzheimer's had the highest levels of amyloid deposits at the start of the study and over time showed a loss of volume in the hippocampal area of the brain.[229] In our rodent studies we measured the BDNF content in the hippocampus, a key brain area involved in learning and memory, and found that it correlated with cognitive function, meaning, when levels of BDNF decreased, so did cognitive function. BDNF has been reported to be reduced in brains from Alzheimer's patients. Whether the decrease in BDNF is related to the accumulation of amylin or not is still unknown.

So where does the amylin come from that accumulates in the brain? As explained in Chapter 4, amylin is produced in the pancreas along with insulin, and the accumulation of amyloid deposits are known to induce apoptosis in pancreatic beta cells. Some of the amylin is also released into the circulation and makes it way to the brain. In the brain, cells have amylin

---

[229] Archives of Neurology, 2009; 66 (12): 1469.

receptors that respond to amylin signaling to reduce food intake and increase metabolism that helps to control body weight. Excessive accumulation of amylin leads to the formation of amyloid plaques. This may provide the link between type 2 diabetes and Alzheimer's, as suggested in the National Institutes of Health report. In addition to the amylin that is produced in the pancreas and enters the blood stream to make its way to the brain, a similar protein known as beta amylin is produced by cells in the brain and accumulates in Alzheimer's disease. We have recently measured serum amylin levels in overweight/obese individuals attending the Pritikin Program and have shown that along with a reduction in fasting insulin, amylin was also reduced by 30 percent in just two weeks.[230] The reduction in serum amylin levels in response to the Pritikin Program could be the result of lowering the refined sugar content of the diet or lowering the saturated fat, both of which induce the pancreatic beta cells to produce more amylin. Whether it is simply a high concentration of amylin or some other factor that is responsible for the formation of amyloid plaques in the pancreas and/or brain is unknown. Amylin in high concentration has been shown in cell culture experiments to induce cell death in both pancreatic beta cells and brain hippocampal cells. Collectively, however, these data suggest that lifestyle may be an important contributor to the development of Alzheimer's.

Scientists from Rush University Medical Center in Chicago predict that the incidence of dementia/Alzheimer's will triple over the next 40 years[231] and put a tremendous strain on the health care systems. They point out that available drugs to treat dementia have only small effects and do not alter disease progression. At the present time the best approach is risk

---

[230] American Journal of Physiology: Endocrinology and Metabolism, 2012; 303: E542.
[231] Neurology, 2013; 80 (19): 1778.

reduction by lifestyle modification. Specifically reducing cardiovascular risk factors including hypertension, diabetes, and obesity as well as modifying health behaviors including smoking, lack of regular exercise, and lack of mental activity might substantially reduce the risk for dementia/Alzheimer's. Reducing chronic low-level inflammation by reducing dietary saturated fats while adding omega-3 fats to the diet should also help. The best advice would be to adopt the Pritikin Program and keep mentally active!

Chapter 8

Summary and Pritikin Program Description

In the preceding chapters the most common and serious diseases found in the Westernized countries and the current theories on how they develop are discussed. An abundance of data suggests that the typical Western lifestyle of inactivity combined with a high-fat, refined-sugar, refined-carbohydrate diet with excess calories is a major contributing factor. These things are summarized in Figure 8.1. It is obvious from the figure arrows that there are many interactions/relationships between the

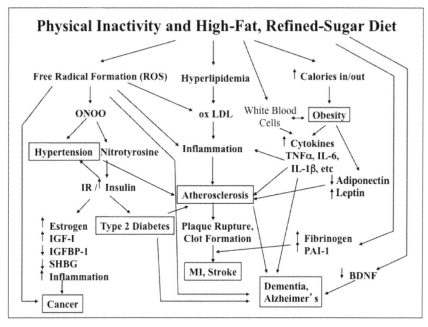

Figure 8.1 Summary of how lifestyle factors relate to the development of common Western diseases.

various causal factors and diseases; in fact, there are many more interactions not indicated due to space limitations. However, the bottom line is the underlying cause – Western lifestyle. The three most prominent factors resulting from the Western lifestyle that seem to underlie many of the health problems are excessive formation of free radicals (reactive oxygen species), chronic production of inflammatory cytokines, especially by white blood cells and fat cells, and the development of hyperinsulinemia. Also discussed in these chapters is the evidence indicating that the Pritikin Program of daily exercise combined with a low-fat, high-fiber, complex-carbohydrate diet of natural foods (not processed) is effective for the prevention and/or treatment of most of these problems.

In addition, the Pritikin Program controls many of these health problems without the need for medication.[232] This is an important point. Unfortunately, many in the pharmaceutical industry through all of its advertising and control of medical research have led society to believe that pills are the answer to most of the health problems presented in Figure 8.1. Medications, in most cases, only treat symptoms, not the true underlying cause of the disease. The benefits of medication have been over exaggerated and most medications have adverse side effects, many of which significantly reduce the quality of life. For individuals who believe that the answer to the health problems so common in Western society is simply taking pills, I suggest you read *Overdosed America* by John Abramson, M.D., who points out that in many cases, lifestyle change is far better than any medication for preventing and/or controlling disease.[233]

The Pritikin Program

The present Pritikin Program is described in Figure 8.2. The core of the Pritikin Program includes daily exercise and the

---

[232] Journal of Applied Physiology, 2005; 98: 3.
[233] Abramson, John. Overdosed America: The Broken Promise of American Medicine. New York: HarperCollins, 2004.

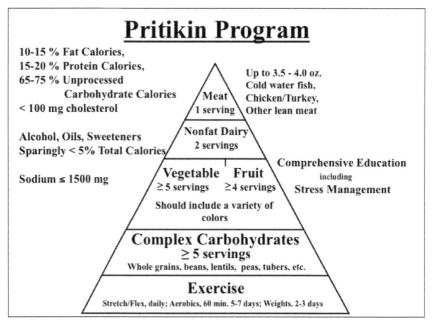

Pritikin Program

10-15 % Fat Calories,
15-20 % Protein Calories,
65-75 % Unprocessed
   Carbohydrate Calories
< 100 mg cholesterol

Alcohol, Oils, Sweeteners
Sparingly < 5% Total Calories

Sodium ≤ 1500 mg

Meat
1 serving

Up to 3.5 - 4.0 oz.
Cold water fish,
Chicken/Turkey,
Other lean meat

Nonfat Dairy
2 servings

Comprehensive Education
including
Stress Management

Vegetable   Fruit
≥ 5 servings   ≥ 4 servings
Should include a variety of
colors

Complex Carbohydrates
≥ 5 servings
Whole grains, beans, lentils, peas, tubers, etc.

Exercise
Stretch/Flex, daily; Aerobics, 60 min. 5-7 days; Weights, 2-3 days

Figure 8.2 Description of the Pritikin Program offered at the Pritikin Longevity Center and Spa in Florida.

Pritikin Eating Plan. In addition to the eating and exercise components, the program at the Pritikin Longevity Center includes a comprehensive educational program with stress management lectures. This book is meant to complement the Center's educational program.

Exercise

The exercise program offered at the Pritikin Center and recommended to be followed at home (Figure 8.2) consists of daily stretching and flexibility exercises, cardiovascular aerobic activities 5-7 days each week, and resistance/weight training 2-3 days each week. These recommendations are consistent with the recommendations of the American College of Sports Medicine/American Heart Association joint exercise report.[234]

---

[234] Medicine & Science in Sports & Exercise, 2007; 39: 1423.

Daily stretching and flexibility activities are especially important for older individuals to keep their joints limber and help to avoid injuries during daily activities such as lifting objects. These activities are especially important for the lower back as many back injuries in older individuals result from tight muscles being used for improper lifting. These activities may also be used as a warm-up and cool-down prior to and after more vigorous sports activities to help avoid injuries. Stretching and flexibility activities should include all of the major muscles in the body. Slowly stretch the muscles and hold for a count of at least 20, then release. Do not bounce or over-stretch the muscles. If you do not have access to a trainer, health club, or coach, there are several good books on stretching by Bob Anderson.

Aerobic cardiovascular activities take the most time. They build endurance, burn calories, and reduce the risk for many health problems including heart disease, cancer, diabetes, hypertension, and other problems, as detailed in the previous chapters. Pritikin recommends 60 min. 5-7 days per week. The standard recommendation from the ACSM/AHA report as well as a report from the Centers for Disease Control and Prevention is for 30 min. of moderately intense exercise 5 days/week to maintain health and reduce the risk for chronic disease. Moderate-intense exercise is defined as working hard enough to raise the heart rate and break a sweat, yet still being able to carry on a conversation. The report also states that 20 min. 3 days/week of vigorous exercise is sufficient for prevention. The ACSM/AHA report also states that to lose weight or maintain weight loss, 60 – 90 min. of aerobic exercise may be necessary, which is consistent with the recommendation from the Institute of

Medicine, National Academy of Sciences, and the Pritikin recommendation.[235, 236] Aerobic cardiovascular activities are exercises that use the large muscle groups in a continuous, rhythmic fashion and include activities such as walking, jogging, cycling, swimming, stair climbing, etc. For older individuals or individuals with health problems, walking is probably the best activity as it takes no special equipment, only comfortable shoes and clothing. If you do have health issues, you should check with your physician before starting any exercise program, especially aerobic cardiovascular activities. Aerobic cardiovascular activities should start out slowly to give the heart a chance to warm up and increase coronary blood flow before more strenuous activity. This is especially important for individuals with heart problems as sudden strenuous activity could precipitate an arrhythmia (irregular heart beat) and heart attack.[237]

The Pritikin Program recommends resistance/weight training 2 – 3 days/week, which is consistent with the ACSM/AHA report. For many years weight training was not recommended for individuals with cardiovascular problems, but that recommendation has been dropped and now weight training is also recommended to cardiac patients.[238] Weight training or resistance exercises are important for maintaining muscle mass -- the calorie-burning tissue in the body. As individuals age, they generally lose muscle mass due to a lack of physical activity and hormonal changes in the body. This is especially true in women and leads to a condition called sarcopenia, where there is

---

[235] U.S. Department of Health and Human Services. Physical Activity and Health: A Report of the Surgeon General. Atlanta, GA: U.S. Department of Health and Human Services, Centers for Disease Control and Prevention, National Center for Chronic Disease Prevention and Health Promotion, 1996.
[236] National Research Council. Dietary Reference Intakes for Energy, Carbohydrate, Fiber, Fat, Fatty Acids, Cholesterol, Protein, and Amino Acids (Macronutrients). Washington, DC: The National Academies Press, 2005.
[237] New England Journal of Medicine, 1993; 329: 1677.
[238] Circulation, 2003; 107: 3109.

generally a loss of muscle fibers and an infiltration of fat into the muscle. This condition causes weakness and frailty and can result in falls. Studies have shown that even individuals in their 90s can benefit from weight training to build muscle and increase strength.[239] Resistance or weight training might include calisthenics, free weights, elastic resistance bands (available in sports equipment stores nationwide), or use of a variety of resistance machines available at most health clubs. These exercises are usually done in sets of 3 using 10, 8, 6 or a similar number of repetitions. Pick a weight you can lift comfortably for the 3 sets and then increase the weight as you get stronger. Resistance/weight training is important for women as well as men. Women don't have to worry about getting muscle bound as they don't have testosterone, but they will get stronger, leaner, more toned, and healthier.

Pritikin Eating Plan

The Pritikin Eating Plan is described as a primarily plant-based diet low in fat, cholesterol, and salt, and high in fiber and a variety of antioxidants. It is really not a diet that one goes on to lose a few pounds, but rather it is a lifetime eating plan for healthy living and disease prevention. In order to avoid many of the common diseases found in the Westernized countries (Figure 8.1), one has to dramatically reduce fat consumption. The Pritikin Eating Plan provides only 10 – 15 percent of calories from fat compared to the typical Western-style intake of 30 – 40 percent or higher. This reduction in fat consumption is achieved by avoiding the use of added oils (in salad dressings or cooking) and by restricting the consumption of animal meat and other animal products, i.e., dairy. Dairy products are limited to 2 servings of nonfat dairy per day, such as nonfat milk, yogurt, or cheese. Nonfat dairy is a good source of calcium but still contains

---

[239] Sports Medicine, 2004; 34: 329.

cholesterol and high-quality protein that can contribute to excess calcium excretion linked to osteoporosis, and increased serum IGF-I, which is linked to cancer. The other aspect of the Pritikin Eating Plan that reduces fat consumption is restricting the consumption of meat to only one serving per day and only up to 3.5 – 4.0 oz; that's about the size of a standard deck of cards, not a Las Vegas deck. The Pritikin Longevity Center diet includes 3 days per week that are strictly vegetarian with no animal meat. Restricting the consumption of animal meat and other animal products keeps the average daily cholesterol consumption to less than 100 mg., the maximum amount the body can handle in most cases. This restriction in the consumption of both fat, especially saturated fat, and cholesterol is responsible for the dramatic reductions in serum cholesterol observed in Pritikin Program participants, usually 20 – 40 percent observed in as little as 3 weeks at the Center.[240] Trans fats that also raise cholesterol are not found on the Pritikin Eating Plan as they are only found in processed foods. Restricting fat consumption (including oils) is very important for weight loss and maintaining a healthy weight. Remember: fat contains 9 calories/gram vs only 4 calories/gram for carbohydrates and protein. Alcohol contains 7 calories/gram, thus limiting alcohol intake is also important for weight loss. At the Center wild cold-water fish (3.5 oz.) is served 3 days/week to increase the intake of omega-3 fatty acids, which is important for reducing chronic low-grade inflammation related to many different common health problems. Please note that I emphasized wild cold-water fish. Salmon, for example, that are farmed may be fed grains and thus do not have as high omega-3 fatty acid content as wild salmon and may also contain high amounts of pesticides.

The bulk of the Pritikin Eating Plan focuses on unrefined complex carbohydrates, vegetables and fruits. Complex

---

[240] Archives of Internal Medicine, 1991; 151: 1389.

carbohydrates (≥ 5 servings per day) include the many whole grains (wheat, rice, barley), beans of various kinds, lentils, peas, and tubers. Vegetables (≥ 5 servings per day) and fruits (≥ 4 servings per day) make up the rest of the diet and should include a variety of colors. The different colors of fruits and vegetables indicate different kinds of antioxidants in the foods. These foods are also low or moderately low in calorie density, and naturally high in fiber, which has many health and weight control benefits. The number of servings above the minimum recommended will depend upon whether or not you need to lose weight and/or how much activity you engage in on a daily basis.

In addition to substantially restricting fat and cholesterol consumption, the Pritikin Eating Plan severely restricts salt intake, allowing no more than 1500 mg of sodium per day. While Pritikin was one of the first to recommend a low-sodium diet, this recommendation is now consistent with the recommendation from the Institute of Medicine.[241] Following this recommendation means that one does not use the salt shaker to add salt during cooking or eating. But it is important to realize that most individuals get the majority of their daily sodium not from the salt shaker in their kitchen but from processed foods or foods served in restaurants as sodium is added in high amounts both as a flavor enhancer and preservative.[242] Since the Pritikin Eating Plan consists of only unprocessed or minimally processed foods that are naturally low in sodium, its adoption automatically reduces the intake of sodium. Here's a good example. Corn in its whole unprocessed state, such as an ear of corn, contains just 3 milligrams of sodium. But when you process corn and turn it into, say, a cup of corn flakes, the sodium content can easily

---

[241] National Research Council. Dietary Reference Intakes for Water, Potassium, Sodium, Chloride, and Sulfate. Washington, DC: The National Academies Press, 2005.
[242] Journal of the American College of Nutrition, 1991; 10(4): 383.

shoot up to nearly 300 milligrams óf sodium. The importance of restricting sodium for preventing and/or controlling high blood pressure is discussed in detail in Chapter 3. The Pritikin Center does use oils and/or sweeteners very sparingly for cooking and relies primarily on herbs and spices as flavor enhancers.

The Pritikin Eating Plan

GO – Recommended Foods

- **Choose at least five servings of unrefined complex carbohydrates per day**

  Five or more servings daily of whole grains (wheat, oats, rye, brown rice, barley, quinoa, millet), starchy vegetables (like potatoes, yams, and winter squashes), chestnuts, beans, and peas. A ½ cup serving is about 80 calories. Limit refined grains (such as white bread, white rice, and white pasta) as much as possible.

- **Choose at least five vegetable servings per day**

  Five (preferably more) servings of raw cooked vegetables daily. A serving (1 cup raw or ½ cup cooked) is about 25 calories. Include dark green, yellow, red, or orange vegetables daily.

- **Choose at least four fruit servings per day**

  Four or more servings of whole fruit daily. For most fruits, a serving fits in your hand and is about 60 calories.

- **Choose two calcium-rich foods per day**

  Two servings daily (90 to 100 calories each). Choose from: nonfat milk (1 cup), nonfat yogurt (3/4 cup), nonfat ricotta (1/2 cup), or soymilk (1 cup).

- **Choose no more than one serving of animal protein per day**

  Fish or shellfish are preferable over lean white meat poultry, and choose lean poultry over lean red meat. A serving is about 3-1/2 to 4 ounces cooked or the size of the palm of your hand and the thickness of a deck of cards.

Optimally, limit poultry to no more than one serving per week and red meat to no more than one serving per month. If you prefer red meat weekly, substitute free-range, grass-fed game meat like bison or venison in place of poultry.

Vegetarian options: For maximal cholesterol reduction, choose on most days legumes like beans, peas, and lentils or soy products like tofu instead of lean meat, fish, or poultry.

Go! In Moderation

- **Beverages**

    Water (plain, bottled, low-sodium, mineral), hot grain beverages (coffee substitutes), and non-medical herbal teas (such as peppermint, rosehips, or chamomile), and cocoa powder – up to 2 tablespoons per day (use non-alkali processed)

    If you choose to drink caffeinated beverages, we recommend green and/or black tea over coffee because of tea's many health benefits.

    We also recommend moderation: no more than 400 mg of caffeine daily (the equivalent of about 4 eight-ounce cups of coffee *or* 8 eight-ounce cups of tea).

    If you prefer coffee, do consider your own personal health history, and ask yourself the following questions:

    - Do I have problems that are linked to or exacerbated with coffee consumption, such as gastrointestinal issues like GERD, panic attacks, sleep troubles, or glaucoma? Does drinking coffee trigger the desire for behaviors (like cigarette smoking) that I'm trying to avoid?

- Is coffee such a profound part of my life that it's getting in the way of healthy habits? For example:

Am I "living" on coffee to the point where I'm not eating food, including healthy foods like fruits and vegetables?

Am I living off the "high" from coffee rather than the much healthier "high" from daily exercise?

Am I depriving myself of healthful restorative sleep because of all the coffee I'm drinking?

If you answered "yes" to any of the above, we recommend that you cut down on your coffee consumption, or avoid coffee altogether.

If none of the above applies to you, and if you enjoy coffee, by all means keep enjoying it. Remember to:

1. Make sure your coffee passes through a paper filter.

2. Drink it black or flavored with nonfat milk, soymilk, and/or zero-calorie sweetener.

How much water should I drink?

If you're eating a typical American diet full of dry, salty, and highly processed foods, the oft-quoted "8 glasses a day" is probably necessary. But if you're eating a really healthy diet like Pritikin, full of water-rich fresh foods like fruits and vegetables, you're probably taking in plenty of water. So our advice is very simple. Drink water when you're thirsty. Stop drinking when you're not. If you exercise in a hot humid climate you will need more water, even more than you crave.

- **Egg Whites**

  Limit to 1 to 2 egg whites per day. Egg whites are available in your grocer's case, or simply, on your own, you can separate the yolks from the whites.

- **If your weight is fine**

  Celebrate! Eat as many whole grains, vegetables, legumes (such as beans and peas), and fruits as you want. Enjoy higher-in-calorie density foods such as avocado and nuts, but limit them to keep your weight under control. Limit avocado intake to no more than 2 ounces per day. Limit walnuts, flaxseeds, almonds, pumpkin seeds, pecans, pistachios, sunflower seeds, filberts (hazelnuts), peanuts, cashews, and macadamia nuts to no more than 1 ounce per day.

- **If you want to lose weight**

  Go wild with vegetables. The more vegetables, including dark green, yellow, red, or orange vegetables, the better!

Limit calorie-dense foods such as dried grains (breads, crackers, cold cereals), dried fruits, nuts, and seeds. Avoid refined or concentrated sweeteners. They all pack a lot of calories into very small amounts of food. You'll find it much easier to feel full and satisfied –and curb hunger – if you focus instead on high-water, high-fiber foods like cooked grains (oatmeal and brown rice), vegetables, and whole fruits. You'll eat more – yet weigh less.

Go easy on fruit and vegetable juices because they provide less satiety than whole fruits and vegetables.

- **Calorie-free sweeteners**

  If you choose to use calorie-free sweeteners, choose sucralose (brand name is Splenda) because it has the best safety record. To keep you moving in the direction of a palate that appreciates and prefers the subtler sweetness of fruit, keep your consumption of Splenda moderate – no more than 10 to 12 packets a day.

CAUTION! - The less, the better

While "Caution" foods are not recommended, this list provides direction when food choices are limited.

- **Refined fats and oils**

  Limit the consumption of ALL oils to no more than 1 teaspoon per 1000 calories consumed, especially if you're trying to lose weight, because all refined oils have the highest calorie density of any food or ingredient.

- **Alcoholic beverages**

  Use in moderation or not at all. For women, up to 4 drinks per week, with no more than ½ to 1 drink per day. For men, up to 7 drinks per week, with no more than 1 to 2 drinks per day. A drink is approximately 5 ounces of wine, 12 ounces of beer, or 1-1/2 ounces of 80 proof liquor. Choose red wine over white wine, wine over beer, and either over liquor.

- **Refined or concentrated sweeteners**

  For healthy individuals who choose to use sweeteners, a suggested rule of thumb is a maximum of 2 tablespoons of fruit juice concentrate or 1 tablespoon of other refined sweeteners (such as honey, agave, barley malt, corn syrup, rice syrup) per 1000 calories consumed. None is optimal. Avoid fructose and high fructose corn syrup.

- **Salt and high-sodium foods, condiments**

  Avoid added salt, and highly salted, pickled, and smoked foods. Limit foods that have more than 1 mg of sodium per calorie so as not to exceed 1200 to 1500 mg of sodium per day, depending on age.

- **Refined grains**

  Limit as much as possible foods containing refined grains (such as white pasta, white bread, and white rice).

STOP! - Think about it first

When faced with foods in the "Stop" category, search for choices in the "Go," and, if necessary, "Caution" foods. "Stop" foods, due to their high content of saturated fat, partially hydrogenated fat, cholesterol, and/or sodium, may significantly compromise your personal health goals.

Limit the following choices to less than once per month. None is optimal.

- **Animal fats, tropical oils, and processed refined oils**

  Such as butter, coconut oil, palm kernel oil, lard, chicken fat, palm oil, cocoa butter, chocolate, margarine, hydrogenated and partially hydrogenated vegetable oils, and shortenings.

- **Meats**

  Such as fatty meats, organ meats, and processed meats (hot dogs, bacon, and bologna.)

- **Whole and low-fat dairy**

  All cheese, cream, cream cheese, half-and-half, ice cream, milk, sour cream, and yogurt, unless fat-free and low in sodium.

- **Nuts**

  Coconuts.

- **Salt and Salt Substitutes**

  Potassium chloride.

Additional potassium in supplement (not food) form may be harmful, especially for older people or those with compromised kidney function. Check with your doctor before taking salt substitutes that contain potassium chloride.

- **Miscellaneous**

   Egg yolks, deep-fried foods, non-dairy whipped toppings, rich desserts and pastries, and salty snack foods.

Tips on How to Start the Pritikin Program

Exercise

First, it is important to realize that the human body was not designed to be sedentary and that virtually every system in the body functions more effectively when you exercise regularly. The first secret to a successful exercise program is to set a schedule and stick to it. For example, I do my stretching/flexibility exercises first thing in the morning. When I was younger and participated in more vigorous sports activities like jogging, I also did some stretching immediately before starting the activity as well as when I finished. Tuesday and Thursday afternoons are scheduled to go to the gym for my resistance/strength training (only 20-30 min). My aerobic training, that is now limited to walking in the hills by my house 5-7 days a week, is done in the early evening when I get home from work and have my apple snack. When you first start your aerobic exercise, you may not be able to go for 60 min. depending on your medical condition. Start with 30 min. or less and work up to 60 min. over a few weeks.

The second secret to my commitment for daily exercise is that I have an exercise partner, actually two, my wife and our dog. Having exercise partners will greatly increase the likelihood that you will exercise on a regular basis. Many times when I get home from work, I don't really feel like going to exercise but due to their urging I go and always feel better both physically and psychologically when we are finished.

Pritikin Eating Plan

Eat to be healthy, don't starve yourself to lose weight. Eat 5-6 smaller meals each day including healthy snacks in the mid morning and mid afternoon. Start by reducing the fat, cholesterol, and salt from your diet by reducing your consumption of meat to no more than 3.5-4.0 oz (size of a deck of cards) each day and eventually trying to have a few days each week being purely vegetarian. Eliminate the use of the salt shaker and consumption of processed foods. Count your servings of fruits and vegetables and be sure you consume the minimum amount (total of 9 servings). Most people consume fewer than 5 serving a day for combined fruits and vegetables, so start by adding fruit to your morning breakfast cereal and include a variety of fruits and/or vegetables in your snacks. An abundance of diet information including recipes can be obtained from www.pritikin.com. You will be surprised how easy it is to adopt the Pritikin Eating Plan and how quickly your health and energy level will improve while you lose excess weight.

Commonly Asked Questions

Q: Which is more important: the Pritikin Eating Plan or the exercise portion of the program?

A: Both! The eating plan is more important for some things, such as lowering cholesterol, while exercise is more important for lowering triglycerides. However, both are important for the prevention/control of diabetes and hypertension as well as many other health problems, including heart disease and cancer.

Q: Do I have to do all 60 min of aerobic exercise at one time?

A: No, you might want to break up the 60 min. recommendation into 2 or 3 different bouts. Also, on the days you do your resistance/weight training, you might use circuit training, which means moving from one muscle group to another without resting; you can include the time as aerobic training.

Q: My home physician is worried because my HDL-cholesterol fell while I was at the Center. Is this of concern?

A: Not really, and for several reasons. First, societies that do not have a high incidence of coronary disease because they have a healthy diet and low LDL-cholesterol also have a low HDL-cholesterol. Second, recent research has suggested that HDL *function* is more important than the level of HDL-cholesterol.[243] HDL normally reduces the risk for coronary heart disease by shuttling cholesterol from the artery to the liver for excretion from the body, as well as reducing the oxidation of LDL-cholesterol, as detailed in Chapter 2. But many individuals with coronary heart disease and/or metabolic syndrome have nonfunctional, *pro*-inflammatory HDL. Recent research showed that men entering the Pritikin Program with metabolic syndrome

---

[243] New England Journal of Medicine, 2011; 364: 127.

had pro-inflammatory HDL, but after the program, and a slight drop in serum HDL-cholesterol, their HDL had converted to *anti-inflammatory*.[244] Furthermore, recent trials with drugs intended to raise HDL-cholesterol have been unsuccessful;[245] one was even stopped due to adverse outcomes.

Q: Do you recommend supplements with the Pritikin Eating Plan?

A: If you are following the Pritikin Eating Plan, you probably do not need any supplements to meet the Recommended Daily Allowances (now known as the Recommended Daily Intake) established by the National Academy of Sciences. One exception may be vitamin D, also known as the sunshine vitamin due to the fact that exposure to the sun stimulates the skin to produce vitamin D. Normally, daily exposure to the sun in a short-sleeved shirt for 15-30 min. will be sufficient. We recommend that you have your serum vitamin D levels measured, and if they are low your physician should recommend a supplement. Vitamin D is well known for its important role in bone development, and recent data also suggest it is important for cancer prevention.[246] Another supplement that you may need is omega-3 fatty acids. If you are not consuming wild cold-water fish 2-3 times each week, we recommend a fish oil supplement to get an adequate amount of omega-3 fatty acids.

Q: What are good sources of omega-3 fatty acids?

A: Most cold-water fish contain the long-chain omega-3 fatty

---

[244] Journal of Applied Physiology, 2006; 101: 1727.
[245] New England Journal of Medicine, 2010; 362; 1563.
[246] Vitamin D and Cancer Prevention: Strengths and Limits of the Evidence, http://www.cancer.gov/cancertopics/factsheet/prevention/vitamin-D (June 2010).

acids (EPA & DHA) that have important health benefits. These are served three days each week at the Pritikin Longevity Center. The Pritikin Program recommends that you get 1 – 1.5 gm of omega-3 fatty acids daily (a 3½-ounce serving of cooked cold-water fish like wild salmon has about 1.8 gm of omega-3 fatty acids), so if you do not consume cold-water fish, you should take fish oil supplements. Some seeds (flax) and nuts (walnuts) do contain omega-3 fatty acids, but they are the shorter chain (18 carbon) fatty acids and have to be converted to the longer chain (20 or 22 carbon as found in fish oil) in the body to provide significant health benefits. The conversion is thought to be somewhat inefficient.[247]

Q; Are multi-grain and whole grain foods the same?

A: Not necessarily. There are some foods that contain several grains that are all refined but are advertised as multi-grain to make you think they are healthy. Read the label and be sure the food is whole grain. The first word you want to see in the Ingredient List is "whole."

---

[247] International Journal for Vitamin and Nutrition Research, 1998; 68 (3):159.

Chapter 9

Nathan Pritikin Research Foundation Publications

While some factors affecting health, such as age, gender, and family history, are not controllable, the Pritikin Program is proven to influence, affect, or reverse a multiplicity of diseases, ailments, and conditions, including:

Heart disease

Angina pain

Hypertension

Type 2 diabetes

Metabolic syndrome

Excess weight/obesity

Prostate cancer

Breast cancer

Colon cancer

High cholesterol

High triglycerides

Peripheral artery disease

Benign prostatic hyperplasia

Chronic inflammation

The following publications provide documentation for all of the above.

2013

Roberts, C.K., A. Izadpanah, S. Angadi, R.J. Barnard. Effects of an intensive short-term diet and exercise intervention: Comparison between normal weight and obese children. *Am J Physiol Regul Integr Comp Physiol.* In press 2013.

Roberts, C.K., A.L. Hevener, and R.J. Barnard. Metabolic syndrome and insulin resistance: underlying causes and modification by exercise training. *Compr Physiol.* 3:1-58,2013.

2012

Izadpanah, A., R.J. Barnard, A.E. Almeda, G.C. Baldwin, S.A. Bridges, E.R. Shellman. C.F. Burant, C.K. Roberts. A short-term diet and exercise intervention ameliorates inflammation and markers of metabolic health in overweight/obese children. *Am J Physiol Endocrinol Metab.* 303:E542-E550,2012

2011

Aronson, W.J., N. Kobayashi, R.J. Barnard, et al. Phase II prospective randomized trial of a low-fat diet with fish oil supplementation in men undergoing radical prostatectomy. *Cancer Prev Res.* 4:2062-2071,2011

2010

Aronson, W.J., R.J. Barnard, S.J. Freedland, S. Henning, D. Elashoff, P. Jardack, P. Cohen, D. Heber and N. Kobayashi. Growth inhibitory effects of a low-fat diet on prostate cancer cells: Results of a prospective randomized dietary intervention trial in men with prostate cancer. *J. Urology* 183:345-350,2010

Barnard, R.J. and W.J. Aronson. Exercise for prevention & treatment of prostate cancer – cellular mechanisms. In; Exercise After Cancer Diagnosis: Impact on Health Outcomes and Quality of Life. J. Saxton and A. Daley eds. Springer Publishing, Chapter 8, p. 141-152, 2010.

2009

Soliman, S., W.J. Aronson, R.J. Barnard. Analyzing serum-stimulated prostate cancer cell lines after low-fat, high-fiber diet and exercise intervention. *Evid Based Complement Alternat Med.* Advance Access published on April 17, 2009; doi: doi:10.1093/ecam/nep031

Barnard, R.J. and W.J. Aronson. Benign prostate hyperplasia: Does lifestyle play a role? *Physician and Sports med.* 37:141-146, 2009

2008

Barnard, R.J. Cancer of the Prostate, Benign Prostatic Hypertrophy, Diet and Exercise Intervention. www.Vitasearch.com, May 2008

Kobayashi, N., R.J. Barnard, J. Said, J. Hong-Gonzales, D.M. Corman, M. Ku, N.B. Doan, D. Elashoff, P. Cohen, W.J. Aronson. Effect of low fat diet on development of prostate cancer and the Akt pathway. *Cancer Res.* 68:3066-3073, 2008

Roberts, C.K., R. James Barnard, Ph.D, Daniel M. Croymans, B.S., University of California, Los Angeles. Weight Loss with a Low-Carbohydrate, Mediterranean, or Low-Fat Diet. *New England Journal of Medicine,* 359:2169, 2008

Barnard, R.J., N. Kobayashi, W.J. Aronson. Effect of diet and exercise intervention on the growth of prostate epithelial cells. *Prostate Cancer and Prostatic Diseases.* 11:362-366, 2008

2007

Sullivan S, Klein S. Effect of a short-term Pritikin diet therapy on the metabolic syndrome. *J CardioMetab Syndrome.* 1:308-312,2006

Roberts, C.K., A.K. Chen, R.J. Barnard. Effect of a short-term diet and exercise intervention in youth on atherosclerotic risk factors. *Atherosclerosis* 191:98-106,2007

Dewell, A., G. Weidner, M.D. Sumner, R.J. Barnard, R.O. Marlin, J.J. Daubenmier, P.R. Carroll, D. Ornish. Evaluation of dietary protein and soy isoflavones in relation to serum IGF-I and IGF binding proteins in the Prostate Cancer Lifestyle Trial. *Nutrition and Cancer* 58:35-42,2007

Barnard, R.J., P.S. Leung, W.J. Aronson, P. Cohen, L.A. Golding. A mechanism to explain how regular exercise might reduce the risk for clinical prostate cancer. *Eur J Cancer Prev.* 16:415-421,2007

Barnard, R.J. Prostate cancer prevention by nutritional means to alleviate metabolic syndrome. *Am. J. Clin. Nutr.* 86(suppl):889S-893S,2007

2006

Roberts, C.K., D. Won, S. Pruthi, S. Kurtovic, R.K. Sindhu, N.D. Vaziri, R.J. Barnard. Effect of a short-term diet and exercise intervention on oxidative stress, inflammation, MMP-9 and monocyte chemotactic activity in overweight/obese men with metabolic syndrome factors. *J Appl Physiol* 100:1657-1665,2006

Booth, F.W., M.V. Chakravarthy. Physical activity and dietary intervention for chronic diseases: a quick fix after all. *J Appl Physiol* (Invited Editorial) 100:1439-1440,2006

Chen, A., C.K. Roberts and R.J. Barnard. Effect of a short-term diet and exercise intervention on metabolic and anthropometric parameters in overweight children and adolescents. *Metabolism* 55:871-878,2006

Roberts, C.K., R.J. Barnard, R.K. Sindhu, M. Jurczak, A. Ehdaie, N.D. Vaziri. Oxidative stress and dysregulation of NAD(P)H oxidase and antioxidant enzymes in diet-induced metabolic syndrome. *Metabolism* 55:928-934,2006

Henning, S.M., W. Aronson, Y. Niu, F. Conde, N.H. Lee, N.P. Seeram, R-P. Lee, J. Lu, D.M. Harris, A. Moro, J. Hong, P-S. Leung, R.J. Barnard, H.G. Ziaee, G. Csathy, V.L.W. Go, H. Wang, D. Heber. Bioavailability and bioactivity of tea polyphenols in humans and mice after green and black tea consumption. *J Nutr.* 136:1839-1843,2006

Pantuk, A.J., J.T. Leppert, W. Aronson, J. Hong, R.J. Barnard, N. Seeram, H. Wang, R. Elashoff, D. Heber, L. Ignarro, A. Belldegrun. Phase II study of pomegranate juice for men with rising PSA following surgery or radiation for prostate cancer. *Clin. Cancer Res.* 12:4018-4026,2006

Roberts, C.K., D. Won, S. Pruthi, R.J. Barnard Effect of diet and exercise intervention on oxidative stress, inflammation and monocyte adhesion in diabetic men. *Diabetes Res.* 73:249-259,2006

Kobayaski, N., R.J. Barnard, S.M. Henning, D. Elashoff, S.T. Reedy, P. Leung, J. Hong-Gonzalez, S.J. Freedland, J. Said, D. Gui, N.P. Seeram, L.M. Popoviciu, D. Bagga, D. Heber, J.A. Glaspy, W.J. Aronson. Effect of Altering Dietary Omega-6: Omega-3 Fatty Acid Ratios on Prostate Cancer Membrane Composition, Cyclooxygenase-2 and Prostaglandin E-2. *Clin Cancer Res.* 12:4662-4670,2006

Barnard, R.J., J.H. Gonzalez, M. Liva, T.H. Ngo. Effect of a low-fat, high-fiber diet and exercise program on breast cancer risk factors in vivo and tumor cell growth and apoptosis in vitro. *Nutrition and Cancer* 55:28-34,2006

Roberts, C.K., C. Ng, S. Hama, R.J. Barnard. Effect of a diet and exercise intervention on inflammatory/anti-inflammatory properties of HDL in men with cardiovascular risk factors. *J. Appl. Physiol.* 101:1727-1732,2006

2005

Roberts, C.K., R.J. Barnard, R.K. Sindhu, M. Jurczak, A. Ehdaie, N.D. Vasiri. A high-fat, refined carbohydrate diet induces endothelial dysfunction, oxidant/antioxidant imbalance and

191

depresses NO synthase protein expression. *J Appl Physiol* 98:203-210, 2005.

Barnard, R.J. and W.J. Aronson. Preclinical models relevant to diet, exercise, and cancer. In: Recent Results in Cancer Research (Controversies in Tumor Prevention and Genetics III). H-J. Senn and R. Morant, eds. Springer 2005, 166:47-62.

Roberts, C.K. and Barnard, R.J. Effect of diet and exercise on chronic disease. *J Appl Physiol* 98:3-30, 2005.

Ornish D, Carroll PR, Fair WR, Pettengill EB, Marlin R, Raisin CJ, Dunn-Emke S, Crutchfield L, Barnard RJ, McCormac P, McNight DJ, Fein JD, Dnstrian AM, Weinstein J, Ngo T, Weidner G. Intensive lifestyle changes may affect the progression of prostate cancer. *J Urol* 174:1065-1070, 2005.

2004
Ngo, T.H., R.J. Barnard, T. Anton, C. Tran, D. Elashoff, D. Heber, S.J. Frieedland and W.J. Aronson. Effect of isocaloric low-fat diet on prostate cancer xenograft progression to androgen independence. *Cancer Res.* 64:1252-1254, 2004.

Wegge, J.K., C.K. Roberts,T.H. Ngo and R.J. Barnard. Effect of diet and exercise intervention on inflammatory markers of atherosclerosis in postmenopausal women. *Metabolism* 53:377-381, 2004.

Molteni, R.A., Wu, S. Vaynmam, R.J. Barnard and F. Gomez-Pinilla. Voluntary physical activity compensates for the deleterious effects of a high-fat, refined-sugar diet on behavioral and neuronal plasticity. *Neuroscience* 123:429-440, 2004.

Leung, P-S.,W.J. Aronson,T.H. Ngo, L.A. Golding and R.J. Barnard. Exercise alters the IGF axis in vivo and increases p53 protein in prostate tumor cells in vitro. *J. Appl. Physiol.* 96:450-454, 2004.

Roberts, C.K., K. Liang, R.J. Barnard, C.H. Kim and N.D. Vaziri. HMG-CoA reductase, cholesterol 7α-hydroxylase, LDL receptor, SR-B1, and ACAT in diet-induced syndrome X. *Kidney International* 66:1503-1511, 2004.

Barnard, R.J. and Aronson, W.J. Diet, Exercise and Prostate Cancer. In: Prostate Cancer, J.N. Lucas ed. Nova Science, Hauppauge, N.Y. Chapter I, 2004.

Barnard, R.J. Prevention of cancer through lifestyle changes. *eCAM Jol* 1:233-239, 2004.

2003

Ngo, T.H., R.J. Barnard, P. Cohen, S. Freedland, C. Tran, F. deGregorio, Y.I. Elshimal, D. Heber and W.J. Aronson. Effect of isocaloric low-fat diet on human LAPC-4 prostate xenografts and the IGF axis in SCID mice. *Clin. Cancer Res* 9:2734, 2003.

Roberts, C.K. and R.J. Barnard. Low-carbohydrate diets as compared with low-fat diets. *New Engl J Med* 349:1000, 2003.

Barnard, R.J. and J.O. Holloszy. The metabolic systems: Aerobic metabolism and substrate utilization in exercising skeletal muscle. in: The History of Exercise Physiology. C.M. Tipton editor, Oxford Press, New York, NY. p 292-320, 2003.

Roberts, C.K., N.D. Vaziri, R.K. Sindhu and R.J. Barnard. A high-fat, refined carbohydrate diet affects renal NO synthase protein expression and salt sensitivity. *J Appl. Physiol* 94:941-946, 2003.

Masley, S., J.J. Kenney and J.S. Novick. Optimal diets to prevent heart disease. *JAMA* 289:1510, 2003.

Barnard, R.J., T.H. Ngo, W.J. Aronson and L.A. Golding. A low-fat diet and/or strenuous exercise alters the IGF axis *in vivo* and reduces prostate tumor cell growth *in vitro*. *Prostate* 56:201-206, 2003.

Ngo, T.H., R.J. Barnard, P. Cohen and W.J. Aronson. IGF-1 and Insulin-like growth factor binding protein-1 (IGFBP-1) modulate prostate cancer cell growth and apoptosis: Possible mediators for the effects of diet and exercise on cancer cell survival. *Endocrinology* 144:2319-2324, 2003.

2002

Roberts, C.K., N.D. Vaziri, and R.J. Barnard. Effect of diet and exercise intervention on blood pressure, insulin oxidative stress, and nitric oxide availability. *Circulation* 106:2530-2532, 2002.

Roberts, C.K., R.J. Barnard, K.H. Lui and N.D. Vaziri. Effect of diet on adipose tissue and skeletal muscle VLDL receptors and

LPL: Implications for obesity and hyperlipidemia. *Atherosclerosis* 161:133-141, 2002.

Roberts. C.K., N.D. Vaziri, Z. Ni, X.Q. Wang and R.J. Barnard. Correction of long-term diet-induced hypertension and protein nitration by diet modification. *Atherosclerosis* 163:321-327, 2002.

Molteni, R., R.J. Barnard, Z. Ying, C.K. Roberts and F. Gomez-Pinilla. A high-fat, refined-sugar diet reduces BDNF, neuronal plasticity, and cognitive function. *Neuroscience* 112:803-814, 2002.

Tymchuk, C.N., R.J. Barnard, T.H. Ngo and W.J. Aronson. The role of testosterone, estradiol, and insulin in diet and exercise-induced reductions in prostate cancer cell growth. *Nutrition and Cancer* 42:112-116, 2002.

Roberts, C.K., J.J. Berger and R.J. Barnard. Long-term effects of diet on leptin, energy intake and activity in a model of diet-induced obesity. *J. Appl. Physiol.* 93:887-893, 2002.

Ngo, T.H., R.J. Barnard, C.N. Tymchuk, P. Cohen. and W.J. Aronson. Effect of diet and exercise on serum insulin, IGF-1, and IGFBP-1 levels and growth of LNCaP cells *in Vitro*. *Cancer Causes & Control* 13:929-935, 2002.

Barnard, R.J., W.J. Aronson, C.N. Tymchuk and T.H. Ngo. Prostate cancer: Another aspect of the insulin resistance syndrome. *Obesity Rev* 3:303-308, 2002.

Barnard, R.J. and J.O. Holloszy. The metabolic systems: Aerobic metabolism and substrate utilization in exercising skeletal muscle. in: The History of Exercise Physiology. C.M. Tipton editor, Oxford Press, New York, NY. p 292-320, 2002.

2001

Roberts, C.K., N.D. Vaziri and R.J. Barnard. Effects of estrogen on gender specific development of diet-induced hypertension. *J. Appl Physiol.* 91:2005-2009, 2001.

Roberts, C.K., N.D. Vaziri, K.H. Liag and R.J. Barnard. Reversibility of long-term diet induced insulin resistance and metabolic syndrome characteristics. *Hypertension* 37:1323-1328, 2001.

Youngren, J.F., J. Paik and R.J. Barnard. Impaired insulin receptor autophosphorylation is an early defect in fat-fed, insulin-resistant rats. *J. Appl. Physiol.* 91:2240-2247, 2001.

Tymchuk, C.N., S.B. Tessler and R.J. Barnard. Changes in sex hormone-binding globulin, insulin and serum lipids in postmenopausal women on a low-fat, high-fiber diet combined with exercise. *Nutrition and Cancer* 38:158-162, 2000.

Tymchuk, C.N., R.J. Barnard, D. Heber and W.J. Aronson. Evidence for an inhibitory effect of diet and exercise on prostate cancer cell growth. *J. Urol.* 166:1185-1189, 2001.

2000

Barnard, R.J. American College of Sports Medicine Position Stand on Exercise and type 2 diabetes. *Am. J. Med. Sports* 2:364-367, 2000.

Roberts, C.K., N.D. Vaziri, X.Q. Wang, and R.J. Barnard. NO inactivation and hypertension induced by a high-fat, refined carbohydrate diet. *Hypertension* 36:423-429, 2000.

Fonseca, V., A. Dicker-Brown, S. Ranganathan, W. Song, R.J. Barnard, L. Fink and P.A. Kern. Effect of a high-fat-sucrose diet on enzymes of homocysteine metabolism in the rat. *Metabolism* 49:736-741, 2000.

1999

Barnard, R.J. The role of exercise in the detection and treatment of peripheral vascular disease.   In. Exercise and the Heart in Health and Disease. R.J. Shephard and H.S. Miller eds. Marcel Dekker, Inc. New York, N.Y., 1999.

Barnard, R.J. and S.B. Inkeles. Effects of on an intensive diet and exercise program on lipids in postmenopausal women. *Women's Health Issues* 9:155-161,1999.

Reil, T.D., R.J. Barnard, V.S. Kashyap, C.K. Roberts and H.A. Gelabert. Diet induced changes in endothelial dependent relaxation of the rat aorta. *J Surg Res* 85:96-100, 1999.

Berger, J.J. and R.J. Barnard. Effect of diet on fat cell size and hormone sensitive lipase activity. *J Appl Physiol.* 87:227-232, 1999.

Barnard, R.J. A carbohydrate diet to prevent and control coronary heart disease. Pritikin was Right. *ACSM's Health and Fitness J.* 3:23-26, 1999.

Roberts, C.K., R.J. Barnard, A. Jasman and T.W. Balon. Acute exercise increases nitric oxide synthase activity in skeletal muscle. *Am J Physiol* 277 (Endocrinol. Metab 40) E390-E394, 1999.

Kenney, J.K., R.J. Barnard and S. Inkeles. Very-low-fat diets do not necessarily promote small, dense LDL particles. *Am J Clin Nutr.* 70:423, 1999.

Barnard, R.J. and S.B. Inkeles. The value of lifestyle change in treating coronary disease - what does it take? *Preventive Cardiology* 2:159-163, 1999.

Barnard, R.J. Very-low-fat diets. *Circulation* 100:1012-1013, 1999.

1998

Barnard, R.J., C.K. Roberts, S.M. Varon and J.J. Berger, Diet-induced insulin resistance precedes other aspects of the metabolic syndrome. *J Appl Physiol,* 84:1311-1315, 1998.

Tymchuk, C.N., S.B. Tessler, W.J. Aronson and R.J. Barnard, Effects of diet and exercise on insulin, sex hormone-binding globulin and prostate-specific antigen. *Nutrition and Cancer,* 31:127-131, 1998.

1997

Barnard, R.J., J.F. Youngren and S.H. Scheck, Reversibility of diet-induced skeletal muscle insulin resistance. *Diabetes Res,* 32:213-221, 1997.

Barnard, R.J., S.C. DiLauro and S.B. Inkeles, Effects of intensive diet and exercise intervention in patients taking cholesterol-lowering drugs. *Am J Cardiol* 79:1112-1114, 1997.

Roberts, C.K., R.J. Barnard, S.H. Sheck and T. W. Balon, Exercise-stimulated glucose transport in skeletal muscle is nitric oxide dependent. *Am J Physiol* 273:E220-E225, 1997.

1996

Beard, C.M., R.J. Barnard, D.C. Robbins, J.M. Ordovas and E.J. Schaefer, Effects of diet and exercise on qualitative and quantitative measures of LDL and its susceptibility to oxidation. *Arterioscler Thromb Vasc Biol,* 16:201-207, 1996.

1995

Bagga, D., J.M. Ashley, S.P. Geffrey, H-J. Wang, R.J. Barnard, S. Korenman and D. Heber, Effects of a very low fat, high fiber diet on serum hormones and menstrual function: Implications for breast cancer prevention. *Cancer,* 76:2491-2496, 1995.

Zernicke, R.F., G.J. Salem, R.J. Barnard, J.S. Woodward Jr., J.W. Meduski and J.D. Meduski, Adaptations of immature trabecular bone to exercise and augmented dietary protein. *Med Sci Sports Exer,* 27:1486-1493, 1995.

Li, K-C, R F. Zernicke, R.J. Barnard and A.F-Y. Li, Response of immature diabetic bone-ligament junctions to insulin and exercise. *Clin Biomech,* 10:331-336, 1995.

Barnard, R.J., J.F. Youngren and D.A. Martin, Diet, not aging causes skeletal muscle insulin resistance. *Gerontology,* 41:205-211, 1995

Czernin, J., R.J. Barnard, K.T. Sun, J. Krivokapich, E. Nitzsche, D. Dorsey, M.E. Philps and H.R. Schelbert, Effect of short-term cardiovascular conditioning and low-fat diet on myocardial blood flow and flow reserve. *Circulation,* 92:197-204, 1995.

Zernicke, R.F., G.J. Salem, R J. Barnard and E. Schramm, Long-term, high-fat-sucrose diet alters rat femoral neck and vertebral morphology, bone mineral content, and mechanical properties. *Bone,* 16:25-31, 1995.

Youngren, J.F. and R.J. Barnard, Effects of acute and chronic exercise on skeletal muscle glucose transport in aged rats. *J Appl Physiol,* 78,1750-1756, 1995.

1994

Barnard, R.J., T. Jung and S.B. Inkeles, Diet and exercise in the treatment of NIDDM - the need for early emphasis. *Diabetes Care,* 17:1469-1472, 1994.

Bagga, D., J.M. Ashley, S. Geffrey, Hei-Jung, R.J. Barnard, R. Elashoff and D. Heber, Modulation of serum and breast duct fluid lipids by a very low-fat, high-fiber diet in premenopausal women. *JNCI,* 86:1419-1421, 1994.

Barnard, R.J. and, S.J. Wen, Exercise and diet in the prevention and control of the metabolic syndrome. *Med Sports* 18:218-228, 1994.

Barnard, R.J., Physical activity, fitness and claudication. In Physical Activity, Fitness and Health 1992 Proceedings. C. Bouchard, R.J. Shephard and T. Stephens, eds. Human Kinetics, Champaign, IL. p 622-632, 1994.

1993

Li, K.C., R. F. Zernicke, R.J. Barnard, A.F.X. Li and P. Campbell. Effects of mild diabetes on immature cortical bone. *Clin Biomech,* 8:49-51, 1993.

Barnard, R.J., D.J. Faria, J.E. Menges, and D.A. Martin, Induction of hyperinsulinemia and related atherosclerotic risk factors by a high-fat, sucrose diet. *Atherosclerosis,* 100: 229-239, 1993.

Li, K-C, R.F. Zernicke, R.J. Barnard and A.F-Y Li. Response of immature bone-ligament junction to a high-fat, sucrose diet. *Clin Biomech,* 8:163-165, 1993.

Hou. J. C-H., R.F. Zernicke, and R.J. Barnard. Effects of severe diabetes on immature rat femoral neck. *J Orthop Res,* 11: 263-271, 1993.

1992

Salem, G.J., R.F. Zernicke and R.J. Barnard. Diet related changes in mechanical properties or rat vertebrae. *Am J Physiology,* 262:R318-R321, 1992.

Barnard, R.J., E.J. Ugianskis and D.A. Martin. The effect of an intensive diet and exercise program on patients with NIDDM and hypertension. *J Cardioresp Rehab,*12:194-201, 1992.

Barnard, R.J., L.O. Lawani, D.A. Martin, J.F. Youngren, R. Singh and S.H. Scheck. Effects of maturation and aging on the skeletal muscle glucose transport system. *Am J Physiol,* 262:E619-E626, 1992.

Barnard, R.J. Response to "Letter to the Editor". *Arch Intern Med,* 152:1721-1723, 1992.

Barnard, R.J., E.J. Ugianskis, D.A. Martin and S.B. Inkeles. Role of diet and exercise in the management of hyperinsulenemia and related atherosclerotic risk factors. *Am J Cardiol,* 69:440-444, 1992.

1991

Li, K-C., R.F. Zernicke, R.J. Barnard and A. F-Y Li. Differential response of rat limb bones to strenuous exercise. *J Appl Physiol,* 70:554-560, 1991.

Scheck, S.H., R.J. Barnard, L.O. Lawani and J.F. Youngren, D.A. Martin and R. Singh. Effects of NIDDM on the glucose transport system in human skeletal muscle. *Diabetes Res,* 16:111-119, 1991.

Barnard, R.J. Effects of life style modification on serum lipids. *Arch Int Med,* 151:1389-1394, 1991.

Hou, J.C-H., R.F. Zernicke and R.J. Barnard. Experimental diabetes, insulin treatment and femoral neck morphology and biomechanics in rats. *Clin Orthop*, 264:278-85, 1991.

Heber, D., J.A. Ashley, D.A. Leaf and R.J. Barnard. Reduction in serum estrodiol in postmenopausal women given free access to a low-fat, high-carbohydrate diet. *Nutrition*, 7:137-40, 1991.

1990

Barnard, R.J. Use of exercise and diet to fight peripheral vascular disease; *Your Patient and Fitness*, 5:12-16, 1990.

Barnard, R.J., D. S. Kartel, J.F. Youngren and D.A. Martin. Effects of streptozotocin-induced diabetes on glucose transport in skeletal muscle. *Endocrinology,*126:1921-1926, 1990.

Barnard, R.J. Serum lipid reductions achieved with diet and exercise. *New Engl J Med,* 323:16, 1990.

Hou, J.C-H., R.F. Zernicke and R.J. Barnard. High-fat sucrose diet effects in femoral neck geometry and biomechanics. *Clin Biomech,* 5:162, 1990.

Hou, J. C-H, G.J. Salem, R.F. Zernicke and R.J. Barnard. Structural and mechanical adaptations of immature trabecular bone to strenuous exercise. *J Appl Physiol,* 69:1309-1314, 1990.

Li, K-C, R.R. Zernicke, R.J. Barnard and A. F-Y Li. Effects of a high-fat, sucrose diet on cortical bone remodeling and biomechanics. *Calcif Tissue Int,* 47:308-313, 1990.

Mehrabian, M., J. Peter, R.J. Barnard and A. Lusis. Dietary regulation of fibrinolytic factors. *Atherosclerosis,* 84:24, 1990.

1989

Kenney, J., M. Rosenthal, S. Inkeles and R.J. Barnard. Letter to the Editor. *New Engl J Med*, 320: 536, 1989.

Sternlicht, E., R.J. Barnard and G.K. Grimditch. Exercise and insulin stimulate skeletal muscle glucose transport through different mechanisms. *Am J Physiol,* 256: E227-E320, 1989.

Sternlicht, E., R.J. Barnard and G.K. Grimditch. B-adrenergic receptors are not responsible for exercise stimulation of glucose transport. *J Appl Physiol,* 66:2419-2422, 1989.

1988

Barnard, R.J. and J.A. Hall. The role of exercise in the detection, treatment and evaluation of patients with peripheral vascular disease; in Exercise and Modern Medicine: Testing and Prescription in Health and Disease. B.A. Franklin, S. Gordon, G.C. Timmis, eds, Williams & Wilkins, Baltimore, MD., 1988.

Barnard, R.J., J.B. Peter, J. Hall and C. Kinsella. Effects of a short-term diet and exercise program on serum apoproteins. *J Appl Nutr,* 40:5-12, 1988.

Barnard, R.J., R. Pritikin, R. Rosenthal and S. Inkeles. Pritikin Approach to Cardiac Rehabilitation; Rehabilitation Medicine, J. Goodgold, ed., C.V. Mosby Company, St. Louis, MO., 1988.

Grimditch, G.K., R.J. Barnard, L. Hendricks and D. Weitzman. Peripheral insulin sensitivity as modified by diet and exercise training. *Am J Clin Nutr,* 48:38-43, 1988.

Reddy, B. S., A. Engle, B. Simi, L.T. O'Brien, R.J. Barnard, N. Pritikin and E. L. Wynder. Effect of low-fat, high carbohydrate, high-fiber diet on fecal bile acids and neutral sterols. *Preventive Med,* 17:432-439, 1988.

Sternlicht, E., R.J. Barnard and G.K. Grimditch. Mechanism of insulin action on glucose transport in rat skeletal muscle. *Am J Physiol,* 254:E633-E638: 1988.

Whitson, R.H., G.K. Grimditch, E. Sternlicht, S.A. Kaplan, R.J. Barnard and K. Itakura. Characterization of rat skeletal muscle sarcolemmal insulin receptors and a sarcolemmal insulin binding inhibitor; *J Biol Chem,* 263:4789-4794, 1988.

1987
Barnard, R.J., J.A. Hall, A. Chaudhari, J.E. Miller and M.A. Kirschenbaum. Effects of low-fat, low-cholesterol diet on serum lipids, platelet aggregation and thromboxane formation. *Prostaglandins Leukotrienes and Medicine,* 26:241-252,1987.

Barnard, R.J., S. Inkeles and K.A. Foon. Nathan Pritikin's Heart. Nutrition Today, 22:39,1987.

Grimditch, G.K., RJ. Barnard, E. Sternlicht, R.H. Whitson and S.A. Kaplan. Effect of diet on insulin binding and glucose transport in rat sarcolemmal vesicles. *Am J Physiol,* 252: E420-E425, 1987.

1986

Grimditch, G.K., R.J. Barnard, S.A. Kaplan and E. Sternlicht. Effect of training on insulin binding to rat skeletal sarcolemmal vesicles. *Am J Physiol,* 250: E570-E575, 1986.

Holly, R G., R.J. Barnard, M. Rosenthal, E. Applegate and N. Pritikin. Triathlete characterization and response to prolonged strenuous competition. *Med Sci Sports Exerc,* 18:123-127, 1986.

1985

Barnard, R.J., J.A. Hall and N. Pritikin. Effects of diet and exercise on blood pressure and viscosity in hypertensive patients. *J Cardiac Rehab,* 5: 185-190, 1985.

Barnard, R.J. Research at the Pritikin Longevity Center. *J Applied Cardiol,* Nov/Dec: 8-12, 1985.

Giardina, S.L., R.W. Schroff, C.S. Woodhouse, D.W. Golde, R.K. Oldham, M.L. Cleary, J. Sklar, N. Pritikin and K.A. Foon. Detection of two distinct malignant B cell clones in a single patient using anti-idiotype monoclonal antibodies and immunoglobulin gene rearrangement. *Blood,* 66: 1017-1021, 1985.

Grimditch, G.K., R.J. Barnard, S.A. Kaplan and E. Sternlicht. Insulin binding and glucose transport in rat skeletal muscle sarcolemmal vesicles. Am J Physiol, 249: E398-E408, 1985.

Hubbard, J.D., S. Inkeles and R.J. Barnard. Nathan Pritikin's Heart. *N Engl J Med,* 313:52, 1985.

O'Brien, L.T., R.J. Barnard, J.A. Hall and N. Pritikin. Effects of a high-complex-carbohydrate low-cholesterol diet plus bran supplement on serum lipids. J Appl Nutr, 37: 26-34, 1985.

Rosenthal, M.B., R.J. Barnard, D.P. Rose, S. Inkeles, J. Hall and N. Pritikin. Effects of a high-complex-carbohydrate, low-fat, low-cholesterol diet on levels of serum lipids and estradiol. *Amer J Med,* 78: 23-27, 1985

1983

Barnard, R.J., P. Guzy, J. Rosenberg and L.T. O'Brien. Effects of an intensive exercise and nutrition program on patients with coronary artery disease: a five-year follow-up. *J Cardiac Rehab,* 3: 183-190, 1983.

Barnard, R.J., M.R. Massey, S. Cherney, L.T. O'Brien and N. Pritikin. Long-term use of a high-complex-carbohydrate, high-fiber, low-fat diet and exercise in the treatment of NIDDM patients. *Diabetes Care,* 6: 268-273, 1983.

Barnard, R.J., S. M. Zifferblatt, J. M. Rosenberg and N. Pritikin. Effects of a high-complex-carbohydrate diet and daily walking on blood pressure and medication status of hypertensive patients. *J. Cardiac Rehab,* 3: 839-846, 1983.

Weber, F., R.J. Barnard and D. Roy. Effects of a high-complex-carbohydrate low-fat diet and daily exercise on individuals 70 years of age and older. *J Gerentol*, 38: 155-161, 1983.

1982

Barnard, R.J., L. Lattimore, R G. Holly, S. Cherny and N. Pritikin. Response of non-insulin-dependent diabetic patients to an intensive program of diet and exercise; *Diabetes Care,* 5: 370-374, 1982.

Dintenfass, L. Effect of a low-fat, low-protein diet on blood viscosity factors in patients with cardiovascular disorders. *Med.J Australia,* 1:543, 1982.

Hall, J.A. and R.J. Barnard. The effects of an intensive 26-day program of diet and exercise on patients with peripheral vascular disease. *J Cardiac Rehab,* 2: 569-574, 1982.

Hall, J.A., G.H. Dixson, R.J. Barnard and N. Pritikin. Effects of diet and exercise on peripheral vascular disease. *Physician Sports Med,* 10: 90-101, 1982.

Pritikin, N. Optimal dietary recommendations: a public health responsibility. *Preventive Med,* 11: 733-739, 1982.

1981

Barnard, R.J., F. Weber, W. Weingarten, C.M. Bennett and N. Pritikin. Effects of an intensive, short-term exercise and nutrition program on patients with coronary heart disease. *J Cardiac Rehab,* 1: 99-105, 1981.

Glossary

Amylin is a protein produced mainly in the pancreas and brain. When too much is produced, it aggregates, forming plaques leading to destruction of beta cells and type 2 diabetes. In the pancreas amylin production is increased by insulin and saturated fatty acids. Regulation of amylin production in the brain is unknown but is associated with Alzheimer's.

Antidiuretic hormone (ADH) is also known as vasopressin and has two main functions: retain water and constrict blood vessels to regulate blood pressure. It is produced in the brain and also has some functions in the brain.

Angina is pain that develops when the heart muscle is deficient in oxygen. It occurs mainly in the chest but can shoot down the left arm or up the neck. Some may have a toothache as angina. If not relieved, angina can lead to a heart attack.

Apoptosis is programmed cell death or cell suicide and is a normal function in the body on a regular basis. Between 50 and 70 billion cells die each day due to apoptosis in the average adult. Too little or too much apoptosis can play a role in disease. For example, if apoptosis is suppressed in cancer cells by IGF-I, the tumor will continue to grow instead of receiving the normal signal to die.

Arrhythmia is the term for an irregular heart beat. There are many different types of arrhythmia, some are benign and some are lethal.

Aromatase is an enzyme found in fat cells and many other cells, including the breast. It is involved in the conversion of androgen (testosterone) and other steroid hormones to estrogen. Aromatase inhibitors have been used to treat women with breast cancer.

Atherosclerosis is the accumulation of cholesterol and other material in the artery wall that blocks the artery, reducing blood flow and oxygen delivery to the tissues. The most common site for atherosclerosis development is the coronary arteries, sometimes referred to as coronary heart (CHD) or coronary artery (CAD) disease.

Body mass index (BMI) is calculated from a person's height and weight and provides an estimate of body fatness. For adults a BMI ≥ 25 is considered overweight and a BMI ≥ 30 is considered obese. A person with a BMI below 18.5 is considered to be underweight. Calculating BMI for children and teens up to and including 19 years of age is a bit more complicated as it has to be adjusted for age and sex. The Centers for Disease Control and Prevention website has a program to calculate BMI.

Cell adhesion molecules (CAMs) are proteins produced in the body for the purpose of having cells stick together. They are involved in the development of atherosclerosis by being produced in the endothelial cells of the artery to attract white blood cells to stick to the artery wall so they can be transported into the artery to accumulate oxidized cholesterol. Some of the CAMs reported to be increased in the development of atherosclerosis include Intercellular Adhesion Molecule 1 (ICAM-1), Vascular Cell Adhesion Molecule 1 (VCAM-1), and Selectins.

Deoxyribonucleic acid (DNA) is a molecule that contains the genetic code or instructions used for production and function of all known living organisms and many viruses.

Diabetes is defined as having a fasting blood sugar (glucose) ≥126 mg/dL or a postprandial (following a meal or glucose load test) glucose ≥200 mg/dL Normal fasting blood glucose is 80-100 mg/dL, and the difference between normal and diabetic is referred to pre-diabetic.

Docosahexaenoic acid (DHA) is an omega-3 fatty acid comprised of 22 carbon atoms with 6 double bonds. It is one of the main fatty acids found in maternal milk and fish oil and is important for the prevention of many different health problems.

Eicosapentaenoic acid (EPA) is an omega-3 fatty acid comprised of 20 carbon atoms with 5 double bonds. Like DHA it is found in maternal milk and fish oil and is also important for the prevention of many health problems.

Free Radicals are atoms or molecules that have lost an electron and are highly reactive ionizing radiation. Many of these radicals are necessary for life and are used by body cells to kill invading bacteria. Excessive amounts can lead to cell injury and contribute to many diseases including atherosclerosis, diabetes, cancer, etc. The most common free radicals formed in the body are oxygen radicals known as ROS.

Hypertension is usually defined as a blood pressure ≥140/90 mm Hg and is the most common cardiovascular disease in the U.S. For individuals with diabetes or kidney disease, a value of 130/80 mmHg is used. Normal blood pressure is < 120/80 mm Hg, and the difference between normal and hypertension is referred to as pre-hypertension.

Inflammatory Cytokines are chemicals produced in the body by white blood cells, fat cells and other cells. They are crucial for the body's immune response toward infections and disease invaders. Over production of inflammatory cytokines can contribute to many diseases, including atherosclerosis, diabetes, cancer, etc. One factor that can lead to over production is saturated fat, resulting in chronic low level inflammation.

Insulin-Like Growth Factor-I (IGF-I) is a protein produced in the body primarily by the liver. It is similar in structure to insulin and has some insulin-like actions. IGF-I's primary action is to mediate the effects of growth hormone associated with growth and development. At maturation the blood level of IGF-I falls dramatically but does not completely disappear. In adults insulin can stimulate the production of IGF-I that in turn can stimulate the growth of tumor cells while blocking apoptosis or cell death.

Insulin-Like Growth Factor Binding Proteins (IGFBP-1) is another protein produced by the liver that binds IGF-I and limits its action. IGFBP-1 production responds to nutritional status and the level of insulin. When insulin is low, IGFBP-1 production is high.

Interlukins are cytokine proteins secreted primarily by white blood cells, fat cells, and other cells in the body. Over 25 different interlukins are known to exist in humans. While most are pro-inflammatory IL-10 is anti-inflammatory.

Lipoprotein lipase (LPL) is a protein produced mainly in muscle and fat cells for the purpose of sitting in the capillary wall and extracting fatty acids from the circulation to be used by the cells for metabolism or storage

Matrix metallopeptidase (MMP) is a family of enzymes produced in the body that have a wide range of functions. Their main function is tissue remodeling and they are thought to play a role in heart attacks, cancer metastasis, arthritis development, etc.

Monocytes are one of the types of white blood cells produced in the body and are found in the blood as well as in tissues. They are part of the body's immune system and produce inflammatory cytokines when activated.

Monocyte chemotactic protein (MCP-1) is a protein produced in the body that recruits white blood cells to sites of inflammation resulting from tissue injury or infection. They are important in atherosclerosis development as the white blood cells recruited into the artery wall capture the oxidized cholesterol forming the cholesterol plaque.

Myocardial Infarction is the medical term for a heart attack, which means that heart cells have been deprived of oxygen, die, and will turn to scar tissue.

Nitric oxide (NO) is a gas produced in the body that was discovered in the late 1980s. It only lasts for a few seconds but has many different functions, including relaxation of the artery wall to lower blood pressure, transporting blood glucose into muscle cells, and kidney excretion of sodium. NO is so important for normal body function that the three doctors who made the discovery were awarded the Nobel Prize in Physiology or Medicine in 1998.

Nuclear factor kappaB (NFkB) is a protein complex found in almost all cells and is described as a transcription factor or a master switch that regulates the cellular responses to stress, cytokines, free radicals, UV radiation, oxidized LDL, bacterial or viral antigens, and saturated fatty acids by activating genes to produce inflammatory factors in the cell.

Reactive oxygen species (ROS) are oxygen atoms or molecules that have lost electrons, forming free radicals.

Renin-angiotensin-aldosterone system (RAAS) is a collection of hormones produced in the body that regulate blood pressure by causing constriction of vessels and retaining sodium and water to increase blood volume. Many people with hypertension take drugs to reduce RAAS activity.

Sex hormone-binding globulin (SHBG) is a protein produced mainly in the liver and binds testosterone and estrogen, limiting their biological actions. SHBG decreases with high levels of insulin, growth hormone, IGF-I, and liver fat production.

Toll-like receptors (TLR) make up a family of receptors found in cell membranes and are known as pattern recognition receptors. TLRs recognize molecules that are broadly shared by pathogens but are distinguishable from normal body components. When the body is under attack by bacteria or virus, the TLRs recognize the foreigners and activate the NFkB super switch to induce inflammatory factors. Saturated fatty acids are also capable of activating the TLRs and NFkB switch, resulting in low-level inflammation that contributes to many diseases.

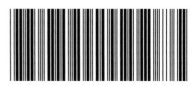